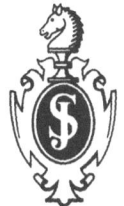

A.H.C. Ratliff · R.M. Atkins · D.M. Eastwood

Selected References in Elective Orthopaedics

With a Foreword by
A. Graham Apley

Springer-Verlag Berlin Heidelberg GmbH

A.H.C. Ratliff, ChM, FRCS
Emeritus Consultant Orthopaedic Surgeon,
United Bristol Hospitals
2 Clifton Park, Bristol BS9 3BS, UK

R.M. Atkins, DM, FRCS
Consultant Senior Lecturer, Department of Orthopaedic Surgery,
Bristol Royal Infirmary, Bristol BS2 8HW, UK

Miss D.M. Eastwood, MB ChB, FRCS
Senior Registrar, Department of Orthopaedic Surgery,
Bristol Royal Infirmary, Bristol BS2 8HW, UK

British Library Cataloguing in Publication Data
Ratliff, A.H.C. (Anthony Hugh Cyril), *1921–*
    Selected references in elective orthopaedics.
    I. Title   II. Atkins, Roger Michael, 1953–   III. Eastwood, Deborah Margaret,
    1957–
    016.6173

Library of Congress Cataloging-in-Publication Data
Ratliff, A.H.C.
Selected references in elective orthopaedics / A.H.C. Ratliff, R.M. Atkins,
D.M. Eastwood.
    p.   cm.
    Includes indexes.
    ISBN 978-3-540-19682-2   ISBN 978-1-4471-1869-5 (eBook)
    DOI 10.1007/978-1-4471-1869-5
1. Orthopedics. I. Atkins, R.M. (Roger Michael, 1953– . II. Eastwood, D.M.
(Deborah Margaret), 1957– .   III. Title.
    [DNLM: 1. Orthopedics–abstracts.   ZWE 168 R236s] RD731.R38 1991
617.3–dc20   91-4928
DNLM/DLC   CIP
for Library of Congress

Typeset by Fox Design, Surbiton, Surrey

2128/3830–543210 Printed on acid-free paper

Foreword

References, to the reader, are like insulin to the diabetic: when needed they are indispensable, but in excess they induce coma. Moreover, when references are simply shovelled into a text in great gobbets, it is hard to resist the suspicion that the author has not read them all, but has copied some from a previous author's list. The story is told of one author who mischievously included in his list a bogus reference to an obscure foreign journal, and gleefully noted its frequent appearance in future articles.

One of the joys of this present book is that the number of references to each topic is very small. But these few have been selected with discretion and studied with care. Each group of references is followed by a critical assessment, written with balanced judgment and commendable brevity, and how refreshing it is to find authors who read much but write little. In fact, these authors have followed the pattern of the sister work, *Selected References in Orthopaedic Trauma*, published in 1989. This is hardly surprising, for that book was widely welcomed, and the two books share the same senior author. Together they constitute an invaluable pair, whose stated objective, to provide the trainee with a small number of authoritative references on important topics, has certainly been achieved. In addition, the selection can help the consultant who is seeking to refresh or deepen his knowledge of any particular topic, and it can provide the research worker with a starting point for probing the literature. Readers will probably regret that the debates which preceded both selection and assessment were not recorded – they must have been highly instructive and enormously entertaining.

The sections into which the book is divided (general orthopaedics, the upper limb, the hand, the spine and the lower limb) reflect the subspecialisation which threatens orthopaedics. Fragmentation and increasingly advanced technology can so easily combine to produce tunnel vision and surgeons whose obsessive concentration on the part leads them to neglect of the whole. But the brevity of this book and the succinctness of each individual contribution help us to retain a sense of perspective.

In the foreword to *Selected References in Orthopaedic Trauma* I wrote that the authors had made one serious mistake, namely that they would not be allowed to rest until they had produced a companion volume on cold orthopaedics. Having completed this new task so splendidly, they probably feel that they can now sit back and relax. Not so – future editions of both books will be demanded. But I suggest a method of lightening their burden. Whenever Journal Clubs meet they should, as part of each session, select one article which could usefully be added to the list of 'Selected References' and, no less important, one which might be deleted. Each substitution must be justified by reasoned argument expressed in a single sentence and sent to Mr A.H.C. Ratliff. Posterity will bless the products.

July 1991   A. Graham Apley

Preface

Following the warm reception of *Selected References in Orthopaedic Trauma,* we felt that there was a need for a companion volume dealing with elective orthopaedics, with a similar aim of selecting authoritative articles on a wide variety of topics.

This book is the result of animated weekly debates over a period of 2 years between three orthopaedic surgeons of differing experience. It does not aim to be comprehensive, but rather presents important papers on controversial subjects, and thus the size of each section tends to reflect the state of current growth and development. Although the final selection of references was our own, where possible we have obtained the advice of experts in each field and we are glad to acknowledge their encouragement and help.

We have cited recent, original articles, and have preferred, where possible, to select from journals which will be readily available to all orthopaedic surgeons. Recent chapters, reviews or monographs have been included if they summarise the current situation. Occasionally an older article has been mentioned if it holds a classic position in the development of a subject. Where necessary we have quoted more obscure references.

Since *Selected References in Orthopaedic Trauma* was produced in 1989, the specialty assessment in orthopaedic surgery has been introduced. A wide knowledge of orthopaedic disease and an awareness of the current literature is expected. During the writing of this volume, we have particularly kept in mind the needs of the candidate approaching this examination and hope to provide a rapid guide to responsible literature. For the established orthopaedic surgeon, the book provides a rapid source of up-to-date information in the management of elective adult and children's orthopaedics.

We are grateful to all our colleagues who have supported this book by suggesting suitable references for inclusion. The manuscript was viii

typed and corrected many times by Mrs Penelope Bull and we are grateful to her for her great expertise and resolute dedication.

Bristol 1991
A.H.C. Ratliff
R.M. Atkins
D.M. Eastwood

Contents

Section 1
General Orthopaedics

Infection

Osteomyelitis

The Classic

Blockey NJ, McAllister TA **Antibiotics in acute osteomyelitis in children** J Bone Joint Surg [Br] 1972;54B:299–309

In 1972, **Blockey** discussed the use of antibiotics in the management of 141 cases of acute osteomyelitis in Glasgow. The opinion was maintained that the correct treatment was rest and antibiotics. Operation was indicated only if pus was detected clinically. The most effective antibiotic combination was fusidic acid and erythromycin. The flora causing the disease was less sensitive to benzylpenicillin than 10 years ago and resistance may develop to methicillin and cloxacillin. Duration of treatment should be 3 weeks.

Acute

McCoy JR, Morrissy RT, Seibert J **Clinical experience with the technetium-99 scan in children** Clin Orthop 1981;154:175–180

Howie DW, Savage JP, Wilson TG, Paterson Sir D **The technetium phosphate bone scan in the diagnosis of osteomyelitis in childhood** J Bone Joint Surg [Am] 1983;65A:431–437

Nade S **Acute haematogenous osteomyelitis in infancy and childhood** J Bone Joint Surg [Br] 1983;65B:109–119

McCoy studied the usefulness of bone scans. The main value in suspected sepsis is to localise affected areas in and around the pelvis and spine. The scan is often unnecessary in the diagnosis of osteomyelitis of long bones. **Howie** debated and defined the value of technetium phosphate scans, based on a study of 280 patients referred with a clinical diagnosis of osteomyelitis. Two groups were compared, with and without definite osteomyelitis. The results indicated that the phosphate scan is highly sensitive and specific in the diagnosis of osteomyelitis in children. In most instances, the scan differentiated focal bone disease from other sites of sepsis, or from non-septic disorders. In 1983, **Nade** reviewed the current controversies of diagnosis and treatment. The subjects debated include the usefulness of radionuclide imaging and its limitations and also the choice and duration of antibiotics. The author presented his indications for surgery, which were the presence of an abscess, the clinical diagnosis of osteomyelitis in a child severely ill and cases with an inadequate initial clinical response to antibiotics. Poor results in the curable disease were due to delay in correct treatment, persistence with conservative treatment and inadequate surgery.

Subacute

Jones NS, Anderson DJ, Stiles P J Osteomyelitis in a general hospital. A 5-year study showing an increase in subacute osteomyelitis J Bone Joint Surg [Br] 1987;69B:779–783

Ross ERS, Cole WG Treatment of subacute osteomyelitis in childhood J Bone Joint Surg [Br] 1985;67B:443–448

Two papers have been included which draw attention to the special problems of subacute osteomyelitis. **Jones** found this type of infection was becoming more widespread, with an insidious onset, lack of systemic symptoms and non-specific radiological changes. Open biopsy and culture were necessary to exclude malignancy. **Ross** divided 71 children with this condition into two groups. In one group, a radiologically "aggressive" lesion required biopsy followed by antibiotics and immobilisation for 6 weeks. In the other, there were cavities in the metaphysis or epiphysis with or without pus. The cause was *Staphylococcus aureus*. With appropriate antibiotics, 91% were cured by a single course of treatment.

Chronic

Kelly PJ Chronic osteomyelitis in adults In: McKibbin B, ed. Recent advances in orthopaedics 4. Edinburgh: Churchill Livingstone, 1983:119–129

Fitzgerald RH, Ruttle PE, Arnold PG, Kelly PJ, Irons GB Local muscle flaps in the treatment of chronic osteomyelitis J Bone Joint Surg [Am] 1985;67A: 175–185

Bjorksten B, Boquist L Histopathological aspects of chronic recurrent multifocal osteomyelitis J Bone Joint Surg [Br] 1980;62B:376–380

Kelly provided a useful general reference to chronic osteomyelitis in the adult based on an experience of 298 cases in the femur and tibia over a 14-year period. He considered there were three objectives in surgical management: removal of dead bone, obliteration of dead space and soft tissue coverage of exposed bone. He advocated the use of external fixation devices to treat unstable infected non-union, and when large soft-tissue and osseous defects remained after debridement of a chronic osteomyelitic lesion. **Fitzgerald** described the application of a local muscle flap to achieve wound closure. With specific antimicrobial therapy, the infection was eradicated in 39 of 42 patients. Various types of cases including infected non-union were discussed. The tibia was involved in 62%, with *Pseudomonas aeruginosa* the most frequently isolated organism. A soleus or gastrocnemius muscle flap was most frequently used. The characteristics of the rare condition of multifocal bone lesions were debated by **Bjorksten**. Twenty patients had a total of 95 lesions; there was a typically prolonged course over several years with varying activity of the disease.

Special Sites

1. Spine

Wenger DR, Bobechko WP, Gilday DL **The spectrum of intervertebral disc-space infection in children** J Bone Joint Surg [Am] 1978;60A:100–108

Eismont FJ, Bohlman HH, Soni PL, Goldberg VM, Freehafer AA **Pyogenic and fungal vertebral osteomyelitis with paralysis** J Bone Joint Surg [Am] 1983;65A:19–29

Discitis, intervertebral disc space infection and vertebral osteomyelitis form a wide spectrum of disorders with a common bacterial aetiology. **Wenger** studied 41 children with symptomatic narrowing of the disc space and fever. Technetium phosphate bone scanning was an accurate and rapid diagnostic tool. **Eismont** discussed the results of treatment in 61 patients with vertebral osteomyelitis. Thirty one had paralysis. Factors which predisposed to the development of paralysis included diabetes, rheumatoid arthritis, increased age and cephalad lesions. For patients with spinal cord compression, the results generally were better with anterior decompression and stabilisation than with laminectomy.

2. Pelvis

Highland TR, LaMont RL **Osteomyelitis of the pelvis in children** J Bone Joint Surg [Am] 1983;65A:230–234

Rosenthal RE, Spickard WA, Markham RD, Rhamy RK **Osteomyelitis of the symphysis pubis – a separate disease from osteitis pubis. Report of three cases and review of the literature** J Bone Joint Surg [Am] 1982;64A:123–128

Pelvic osteomyelitis in children is an uncommon lesion; it is usually thought that the lesion is diagnosed late and that it requires surgical drainage. **Highland** reported 16 cases. The technetium bone scan assisted early diagnosis. In all the patients in this study, antibiotic therapy alone sufficed and surgical drainage was not required. Osteomyelitis of the symphysis pubis is usually preceded by urological or gynaecological surgery and does not respond to short term antibiotic treatment. **Rosenthal** has provided a useful reference for this rare condition. It should be treated by debridement and curettage together with long term high dose antibiotics.

Atypical Bacteriology

Baxter MP, Finnegan MA **Skeletal infection by group B beta-haemolytic streptococci in neonates – a case report and review of the literature** J Bone Joint Surg [Br] 1988;70B:812–814

Hall BB, Fitzgerald RH, Rosenblatt JE **Anaerobic osteomyelitis** J Bone Joint Surg [Am] 1983;65A:30–35

Miskew DBW, Lorenz MA, Pearson RL, Pankovich AM *Pseudomonas aeruginosa* **bone and joint infection in drug abusers** J Bone Joint Surg [Am] 1983;65A:829–832

Baxter studied osteomyelitis in the neonate caused by haemolytic streptococcus. **Hall** drew attention to the incidence of anaerobic osteomyelitis and considered that it was greater than was previously believed. Anaerobic bacteria were isolated from approximately one in four patients where surgical debridement for osteomyelitis was carried out. Mixed aerobic and anaerobic osteomyelitis of long duration has a poorer prognosis than does aerobic osteomyelitis. It is therefore advised that anaerobic cultures should be obtained routinely for all patients with osteomyelitis, so that appropriate antimicrobial therapy can be employed. **Miskew** described experience of 39 sites of *Pseudomonas aeruginosa* bone and joint infection in 35 intravenous drug abusers treated over a 4-year period in Chicago. Awareness of the possibility of this diagnosis is essential. Most patients responded to long term therapy with intravenous aminoglycosides and carbenicillin. Extensive surgical procedures were rarely indicated.

Suppurative Arthritis in the Child

Clinical Studies

Eyre-Brook AL **Septic arthritis of the hip and osteomyelitis of the upper end of the femur in infants** J Bone Joint Surg [Br] 1960;42B:11–20

Wilson NIL, Di Paola M **Acute septic arthritis in infancy and childhood: 10 years' experience** J Bone Joint Surg [Br] 1986;68B:584–587

Morrissy RT, Shore SL **Septic arthritis in children** In: Gustilo RB, Gruninger RP, Tsukayama DT, eds. Orthopaedic infection, diagnosis and treatment. Philadelphia: WB Saunders, 1989:261–270

Review Article

Nade S **Acute septic arthritis in infancy and childhood** J Bone Joint Surg [Br] 1983;65B:234–241

Eyre-Brook reviewed 10 infants with septic arthritis of the hip. Seven showed evidence of osteomyelitis of the upper end of the femur. The various sequelae which may result are illustrated, including destruction of the capital epiphysis and dislocation. **Wilson** discussed a 10-year experience of 61 children with acute septic arthritis. He considered that arthrotomy should be selective rather than mandatory. Septic arthritis of the hip in infants requires arthrotomy, but in the older child an infected hip may be treated by aspiration if the duration of symptoms is short. Infected joints other than the hip can be managed by aspiration. **Morrissy** stated that technetium bone scans do not have the same value in evaluation of joint sepsis as in osteomyelitis. Aspiration of pus from the joint is the first step in treatment. However, cultures are positive in only 60%. In infants, the two most common organisms are *Haemophilus influenzae* type B and *Staphylococcus aureus*. **Nade** stressed the need for effective concentrations of a sensitive antibiotic in the joint. Blood cultures should be performed before antibiotics are administered. Septic arthritis of the hip, particularly in the infant, should be treated by antibiotics and surgical incision and drainage. In other joints, there is still controversy as to whether open drainage should be performed. Repeated aspiration has its advocates.

Tuberculosis of Bone and Joint

Davies PDO, Humphries MJ, Byfield SP, Nunn AJ, Darbyshire JH, Citron KM, Fox W **Bone and Joint Tuberculosis – a survey of notifications in England and Wales** J Bone Joint Surg [Br] 1984;66B:326–330

Davies described the results of a survey of the incidence of bone and joint tuberculosis in England and Wales in a 6-month period in 1978. Of approximately 4000 cases notified, 200 had a bone or joint lesion. More than half of these were of Indian sub-continent ethnic origin. The spine was the most common site. The

Mycobacterium tuberculosis was isolated from the orthopaedic lesions in a high percentage of patients. Drug resistance was rare. (For chemotherapy of tuberculosis, see Tuberculosis of Spine. See individual sections for tuberculosis of the hip and the knee.)

Tumours: Primary

General Principles

Staging

Enneking WF., Spanier SS, Goodman MA **A system for the surgical staging of musculoskeletal sarcoma** Clin Orthop 1980;153:106–120

Biopsy

Simon MA **Current concepts review: biopsy of musculoskeletal tumours** J Bone Joint Surg [Am] 1982;64A:1253–1257

Mankin HJ, Lange TA, Spanier SS **The hazards of biopsy in patients with malignant primary bone and soft-tissue tumours** J Bone Joint Surg [Am] 1982;64A:1121–1127

Radiology

Bloem JL, Taminiau AMH, Eulderink F, Hermans J, Pauwells EKJ **Radiologic staging of primary bone sarcoma: MR imaging, scintigraphy, angiography and CT correlated with pathologic examination** Radiology 1988;169:805–810

Limb-Sparing Treatment

National Institute of Health consensus conference on limb-sparing treatment of adult soft-tissue sarcomas and osteosarcoma JAMA 1985;254;13:1791–1794

Mankin HJ, Doppelt S, Tomford W **Clinical experience with allograft implantation. The first 10 years** Clin Orthop 1983;174:69–86

Review Article

Sim FH **Management of primary malignant tumours of bone** In: Galasko CSB, Noble J, eds. Current trends in orthopaedic surgery. Manchester: Manchester University Press, 1988;48–71

GENERAL ORTHOPAEDICS

Enneking in 1980 described a system of staging of sarcoma: the low-grade lesion without metastases (I), a high-grade lesion without metastases (II) and a lesion of either grade with regional or distant metastases (III). The first two stages are further divided by the anatomical site into either compartmental or extracompartmental lesions. The system stages each tumour according to the risk to the patient. It is more helpful in the assessment and surgical treatment of musculoskeletal sarcomata than other systems and allows comparison of results of various treatment protocols between different centres. **Simon** discussed the crucial importance of biopsy, stressing the operative technique and tissue examination. The skin incision must be carefully planned in order not to compromise subsequent surgery. **Mankin** discussed the hazards based on an analysis of 330 patients from many oncology centres in the USA. There were 18% major errors in diagnosis and 10% non-representative or technically poor biopsies. Problems arose in the skin or soft tissue of the biopsy wounds in 17%. **Bloem** concluded that MR imaging was significantly superior to CT scintigraphy in defining intraosseous tumour length and it was as accurate as CT in demonstrating cortical bone and joint involvement. MR imaging was superior to CT in demonstrating involvement of muscle compartments and it was the modality of choice for the local staging of primary bone tumours. A **consensus conference** in 1984 in the USA provided a summary of current opinions on the principles of management of osteosarcoma at that time, including the extent of surgical resection required and the value of preoperative and postoperative chemotherapy. The paper by **Mankin** in 1983 summarised an experience of 150 resections and allograft implantation for tumours. The grafts performed acceptably in 70% and the results were better in patients with low-grade tumours or benign conditions. **Sim** reviewed recent advances in the management of primary tumours of bone in a concise chapter in 1988.

Osteosarcoma

Goorin AM, Abelson HT, Frei E (III) **Medical progress: osteosarcoma: 15 years later** N Engl J Med 1985;313:1637–1643

Simon MA, Nachman J **Current concepts review: the clinical utility of preoperative therapy for sarcomas** J Bone Joint Surg [Am] 1986;68A:1458–1463

Link MP, Goorin AM, Miser AW et al **The effect of adjuvant chemotherapy on relapse free survival in patients with osteosarcoma of the extremity** N Engl J Med 1986;314:1600–1606

Simon MA **Current concepts review: causes of increased survival of patients with osteosarcoma: current controversies** J Bone Joint Surg [Am] 1984;66A: 306–310

Souhami RL, Craft AW **Annotation: progress in management of malignant bone tumours** J Bone Joint Surg [Br] 1988;70B:345–347

Springfield DS, Schmidt R, Graham-Pole J, Marcus RB, Spanier SS, Enneking WF **Surgical treatment for osteosarcoma** J Bone Joint Surg [Am] 1988;70A: 1124–1130

Simon MA, Aschliman MA, Thomas N, Mankin HJ **Limb salvage treatment versus amputation for osteosarcoma of the distal end of the femur** J Bone Joint Surg [Am] 1986;68A:1331–1337

Goorin summarised progress in the management of osteosarcoma. Before 1972 the 5-year survival rate of osteosarcoma was uniform in many reporting institutions, at about 20%. The outlook for patients with osteosarcoma has improved dramatically in the 15 years since the first trials of adjuvant therapy for the disease. **Simon** explained that in most chemotherapeutic programmes for osteosarcoma, either intravenous or intra-arterial chemotherapy is employed without local radiation therapy prior to the definitive surgical procedure. The results of these differing methods of treatment were reviewed. **Link** reported the results of a randomised controlled trial to determine the value of multi-agent adjuvant chemotherapy based on a study of 36 patients assigned to chemotherapy or observation. He concluded that chemotherapy increased the chance of relapse-free survival of patients with high-grade osteosarcoma, and that it should be given to all such patients. **Simon** (1984) debated the reasons for the increased survival of patients with osteosarcoma. These include earlier diagnosis, meticulous clinical staging procedures, the increased use of thoracotomy for removal of metastases and the employment of limb salvage surgery. **Souhami** summarised progress in the last decade, stressing the trend towards limb conservation in osteosarcoma of the femur, upper tibia and upper humerus. Prosthetic replacement is associated with good functional results, especially in the lower femur, but it poses considerable problems. **Springfield** studied 53 patients who had a high-grade osteosarcoma treated either by resection and limb salvage or amputation. He concluded that when a wide surgical margin can be used and a functional limb salvaged, an amputation is probably not required. **Simon** in 1986 published the results of a retrospective multi-institutional study of 227 patients with osteosarcoma of the distal end of the femur. The overall rate of survival was 55% at 5 years. Compared with above-knee amputation or disarticulation of the hip, the use of a limb salvage procedure did not shorten the disease-free interval or compromise long term survival.

Parosteal Osteosarcoma

Campanacci M, Picci P, Gherlinzoni F, Guerra A, Bertoni F, Neff JR **Parosteal osteosarcoma** J Bone Joint Surg [Br] 1984;66B:313-321

Kavanagh TG, Cannon SR, Pringle J, Stoker DJ, Kemp HBS **Parosteal osteosarcoma: treatment by wide resection and prosthetic replacement** J Bone Joint Surg [Br] 1990;72B:959–965

Forty-one cases of parosteal osteosarcoma were reviewed by **Campanacci**. The adverse significance of intramedullary involvement is stressed. No patients with adequate surgical management and excision developed local recurrence. The special characteristics of this tumour are summarised. **Kavanagh** reviewed 20 cases treated by wide local resection and prosthetic replacement and followed for 6–17 years. Limb function was excellent in 85%. After this mode of treatment, the outcome was not related to medullary invasion by the tumour.

Paget's Sarcoma

Schajowicz F, Araujo ES, Berenstein M **Sarcoma complicating Paget's disease of bone: a clinicopathological study of 62 cases** J Bone Joint Surg [Br] 1983;65B:299–307

Schajowicz reviewed the clinical and pathological features of 62 cases of sarcomatous change in Paget's disease. Most of the sarcomas occurred in polyostotic disease. Tumours often develop simultaneously, or at short time intervals, in the same or different bones. The histological features are characteristic. The prognosis is poor and survival after 5 years is very rare.

Ewing's Sarcoma

Sim FH **Management of primary malignant tumours of bone** In: Galasko CSB, Noble J, eds. Current trends in orthopaedic surgery. Manchester: Manchester University Press, 1988:59–66

Souhami RL, Craft AW **Annotation: progress in management of malignant bone tumours** J Bone Joint Surg [Br] 1988;70B:345–347

Springfield DS, Pagliarulo C **Fractures of long bones previously treated for Ewing's sarcoma** J Bone Joint Surg [Am] 1985; 67A:477–481

Li WK, Lane JM, Rosen G, Marcove RC, Capurros B, Hubos A, Groshem S **Pelvic Ewing's sarcoma. Advances in treatment** J Bone Joint Surg [Am] 1983;65A:738–747

Jurgens H, Exner U, Gadner H, Harms D, Michaelis J, Sauer R, Treuner J, Voute T, Winklemann W, Winkler K, Gobel U **Multidisciplinary treatment of primary Ewing's sarcoma of bone: a 6-year experience of a European cooperative trial** Cancer 1988;61:23–32

Sim debated the controversies of radiation therapy and surgical resection for treatment of Ewing's sarcoma. **Souhami** outlined the improving management of this tumour since chemotherapy has become more effective, and he noted a trend towards surgery for control of the primary tumour. **Springfield** drew attention to the significant risk of fracture of the involved bone in patients with Ewing's sarcoma who survive following irradiation and chemotherapy. **Li** described a study of 18 patients with Ewing's tumour of the pelvis. He suggested that these tumours are best treated by chemotherapy followed by a wide resection and radiotherapy. **Jurgens** reported the results of a 6-year experience of the treatment of 93 patients. The estimated disease-free survival was 60% at 3 years. The local failure rate was high in patients treated with radiation. Tumour volume was a significant factor influencing prognosis. In patients who had surgery for local control, the histological response to chemotherapy had a strong influence on survival. Tumour load and responsiveness to chemotherapy are the two major factors influencing prognosis.

Sarcoma and Joint Replacement

Hamblen DL, Carter RL **Editorial: sarcoma and joint replacement** J Bone Joint Surg [Br] 1984;66B:625–627

Apley AG **Editorial: malignancy and joint replacement: the tip of an iceberg?** J Bone Joint Surg [Br] 1989;71B:1

A few reports have been published where a malignant tumour has developed in bone adjacent to a total hip replacement. **Hamblen** and **Apley** provide references on the controversies in this subject.

Malignant Fibrous Histiocytoma

Souhami RL, Craft AW **Annotation: progress in management of malignant bone tumours** J Bone Joint Surg [Br] 1988;70B:345–347

Capanna R, Bertoni F, Bacchini P, Bacci G, Guerra A, Campanacci M **Malignant fibrous histiocytoma of bone: the experience at the Rizzoli Institute: report of 90 cases** Cancer 1984;54:177–187

Souhami referred to trends in the management of malignant fibrous histiocytoma. The tumour is associated with a 25%–30% 5-year survival when treated with surgical resection alone, but chemotherapy may well improve these results. A detailed study of the results of treatment of 90 patients has been outlined by **Capanna**. Adjuvant chemotherapy was not effective in preventing local recurrence in patients with inadequate surgery.

Chondrosarcoma

The Classic

Henderson ED, Dahlin DC **Chondrosarcoma of bone – a study of 288 cases** J Bone Joint Surg [Am] 1963;45A:1450–1458

Henderson, in a classic paper in 1963, stressed the essential features of this tumour based on a study of a large series from the Mayo Clinic. The tumour presents with a bewildering variety of clinical courses, but if not adequately removed, kills all its victims by recurrence or metastasis. Growth is slow and metastases late.

Review Articles

Gitelis S, Bertoni F, Picci P, Campanacci M **Chondrosarcoma of bone: the experience at the Instituto Ortopedico Rizzoli** J Bone Joint Surg [Am] 1981; 63A:1248–1257

Pritchard DJ, Lunke RJ, Taylor WF, Dahlin DC, Medley BE **Chondrosarcoma: a clinicopathologic and statistical analysis** Cancer 1980;45:149–157

Meachim G **Editorial: histological grading of chondrosarcomata** J Bone Joint Surg [Br] 1979;61B:393–394

Roberts PH, Price CHG **Chondrosarcoma of the bones of the hand** J Bone Joint Surg [Br] 1977;59B:213–221

Gitelis described experience with 125 patients from the Rizzoli Institute. Metastasis and survival were related to the histological grade of the tumour. Adequacy of treatment influenced the incidence of recurrence and length of survival. **Pritchard** studied the case histories and histology of 280 patients. The size and grade of the tumour greatly influenced the prognosis. Metastasis was rare in the absence of local recurrence. Complete ablation of the primary lesion is the treatment goal. **Meachim** reminded surgeons of the difficulties of grading of the histology of cartilage tumours. The paper by **Roberts** is included since it reported a study from the Bristol Bone Tumour Registry, of 19 aggressive cartilage tumours in the bones of the hand.

Soft-tissue Sarcoma

Westbury G **Annotation: the management of soft tissue sarcomas** J Bone Joint Surg [Br] 1989;71B:2–3

Westbury, from his unique experience, has summarised the special problems of management of the rare soft-tissue sarcomas. Although surgical exposure and removal should be radical, as many as one-third can be sterilised by irradiation alone, and radiotherapy substantially improves local control after less than radical resection. For this reason, the consensus has swung away from amputation. The prognosis for surgical treatment is determined by the size and histological grade of the tumour.

Giant-cell Tumour

Goldenberg RR, Campbell CJ, Bonfiglio M **Giant-cell tumour of bone. An analysis of 218 cases** J Bone Joint Surg [Am] 1970;52A:619–664

Sung HW, Kuo DP, Shu WP, Chai YB, Liu CC, Li SM **Giant-cell tumour of bone: analysis of 208 cases in Chinese patients** J Bone Joint Surg [Am] 1982;64A: 755–761

Campanacci M, Baldini N, Boriani S, Sudanese A **Giant-cell tumour of bone** J Bone Joint Surg [Am] 1987;69A:106–114

Goldenberg analysed 218 cases of giant-cell tumour observed for 10 years. This paper provides a comprehensive review of the natural history of various forms of treatment of this rare tumour. There was an overall recurrence rate of 35% and simple curettage alone gave the highest recurrence. More recently, **Sung** noted that giant-cell tumour appeared to be more frequent in the Chinese. The rate of recurrence was lower in patients who were treated by resection and joint fusion. Possible methods of treatment were debated. **Campanacci** studied the results of treatment of 280 cases followed for 2–44 years. Local recurrence usually appeared in the first 3 years after surgery. The factor which influenced the outcome was the surgical margin. There were no recurrences after a wide or radical procedure.

Pigmented Villonodular Synovitis

Rao AS, Vigorita VJ **Pigmented villonodular synovitis (giant-cell tumour of the tendon sheath and synovial membrane): a review of 81 cases** J Bone Joint Surg [Am] 1984;66A:76–94

Rao reviewed 81 patients with pigmented villonodular synovitis and giant-cell tumour of the tendon sheath. The lesion was slow-growing and most common in the fingers and knees. The centrifugal growth pattern and distinct characteristics suggest that this condition is a true neoplastic process.

Synovial Chondromatosis

Maurice H, Crone M, Watt I **Synovial chondromatosis** J Bone Joint Surg [Br] 1988;70B:807–811

Maurice reviewed 53 cases of synovial chondromatosis and compared their clinical, radiological and pathological features. Thirty-nine involved the knee. The disease may be extra-articular or intra-articular. In localised intra-articular disease, metaplasia is confined to one area of the joint and complete excision is curative. A scheme of management is suggested.

Osteoid Osteoma and Osteoblastoma

Healey JH, Ghelman B **Osteoid osteoma and osteoblastoma. Current concepts and recent advances** Clin Orthop 1986;204:76–85

Healey reviewed clinical knowledge of osteoid osteoma stressing that these lesions are common. Preoperative localisation with CT scans has reduced the recurrence rate. Complete excision is successful in eradicating the tumour and removing pain. Osteoblastomas are rare tumours which may achieve a larger size and behave more aggressively than osteoid osteomas.

Bone Cysts

Campanacci M, Capanna R, Picci P **Unicameral and aneurysmal bone cysts** Clin Orthop 1986;204:25–36

Campanacci compared the results of treatment of 178 cases of unicameral bone cysts with curettage and bone grafting, with 141 cases treated with cortisone injections. The end results were comparable in the two groups. The characteristics of aneurysmal bone cysts were discussed based on a report of 198 cases. Radiotherapy is indicated only in inoperable cases.

Chordoma

Mindell ER **Current concepts review: chordoma** J Bone Joint. Surg [Am] 1981; 63A:501–505

Mindell discussed the rare and difficult problem of the diagnosis and treatment of a chordoma, particularly of the sacrococcygeal type.

Pelvic Tumours

Enneking WF, Dunham WK **Resection and reconstruction for primary neoplasm involving the innominate bone** J Bone Joint Surg [Am] 1978;60A: 731–746

O'Connor MI, Sim FH **Salvage of the limb in the treatment of malignant pelvic tumours** J Bone Joint Surg [Am] 1989;71A:481–494

Carter SR, Eastwood DM, Grimer RJ, Sneath RS **Hindquarter amputation for tumours of the musculo-skeletal system** J Bone Joint Surg [Br] 1990;72B: 490–493

Enneking reported experience in 32 patients with pelvic disease and discussed the surgical technique and results. During the last decade there has been a trend towards radical resection of parts of the ilium as opposed to hemipelvectomy. **O'Connor** discussed the operative treatment of 60 patients for a primary malignant tumour of the pelvis. Chondrosarcoma, osteosarcoma and fibrosarcoma were common diagnoses. The best functional results occurred after resection where femorosacral continuity was maintained. Salvage is justified providing a satisfactory margin can be achieved by excision of the tumour. **Carter** reviewed 34 hindquarter amputations performed for malignant tumours around the hip. This article has been selected as a recent source of experience on this subject.

Book Reference

Enneking WF In: Enneking WF, ed. **Muscoloskeletal tumor surgery Vols I and II.** New York: Churchill Livingstone, 1983 (Vol I 494–529, surgical procedures discussing the three major types of pelvic excision).

Tumours: Secondary

General

See **Malignant disease** In: Ratliff AHC, Dixon JH, Magnussen PA, Young SK, eds. Selected references in orthopaedic trauma. London: Springer-Verlag, 1988 Upper limb metastases, lower limb metastases and spinal metastases 12–14

The Spine

See pp. 111–112.

Metabolic Bone Disease

Osteoporosis

Review Articles

Barth RW, Lane JM **Osteoporosis** Orthop Clin North Am 1988;19:845–858

Lindsay R **The management of osteoporosis** In: Baillière's clinical endocrinology and metabolism. Vol 2. 1988; 1:103–124

Barth provided a concise practical update on the aetiology and clinical presentation of osteoporosis. Treatment is both complex and controversial. The value of exercise, calcium supplementation, oestrogen, fluoride and calcitonin are debated. Arresting bone loss has proved to be more effective than rebuilding a depleted skeleton. Every postmenopausal white female up to the age of 65 should be considered immediately for oestrogen replacement therapy aimed at preventing osteoporosis, but the use of oestrogens is not without risks. The goal for the future should be identification of those individuals at highest risk at a young age, before skeletal mass is lost. **Lindsay** debated treatment of the asymptomatic patient with oestrogens, calcium and exercise. Treatment of the established disorder, and particularly with fractures, is more difficult. Special mention is made of fluoride. This remains the only therapeutic agent that stimulates the osteoblast population to begin to synthesise new bone. However, care must be taken in its use and its efficacy has yet to be finally established.

Fractures

The subject of osteoporosis and fractures has been previously considered in **Selected references in orthopaedic trauma** (Ratliff et al 1988; 15–16).

Rickets, Osteomalacia and Osteodystrophy

Mankin HJ **Rickets, osteomalacia and renal osteodystrophy: an update** Orthop Clin North Am 1990;21:81–96

Eisman JA **Osteomalacia** In: Baillière's clinical endocrinology and metabolism. Vol 2. 1988;1:125–155

Kanis JA **Vitamin D metabolism and its clinical application** J Bone Joint Surg [Br] 1982;64B:542–560

Mankin has provided a summary of the subject. Patients with osteomalacia of varying causes may only be distinguished by a biochemical analysis. It is suggested that the orthopaedic surgeon should be aware of the clinical presentation and possible radiographic and laboratory findings. The management has become complex and the realm of the expert physician. The articles by **Eisman** and **Kanis** have been included for detailed reference.

Hyperparathyroidism

Smith R **Parathyroids and bone disease** In: Smith R, ed. Biochemical disorders of the skeleton. London: Butterworths,1979:160–179

Stulberg BN, Licata AA, Bauer TW, Belhobek GH **Hyperparathyroidism, hyperthyroidism and Cushing's disease** Orthop Clin North Am 1984;15: 697–710

Smith discussed the pathology and clinical features of parathyroid overactivity. Osteitis fibrosa presents with bone pain, tenderness, deformity and pathological fractures. Renal calculi are common. When hypocalcaemia is prolonged due to failure of the glomerulus, the parathyroids respond by increasing their activity, resulting in secondary hyperparathyroidism. **Stulberg** described the metabolic bone diseases associated with hyperparathyroidism, hyperthyroidism and hypercortisolism. These diseases cause bone loss which can be treated.

Paget's Disease

Review Articles

Merkow RL, Lane JM **Paget's disease of bone** Orthop Clin North Am 1990;21: 171–189

Kanis JA, Gray RES **Long-term follow-up observations on treatment in Paget's disease of bone** Clin Orthop 1987;217:99–125

Merkow has provided a recent review of the subject. The two major therapeutic agents available for treatment are calcitonins and diphosphonates. The aim of therapy is to control the metabolic activity of the disease and to improve symptoms, especially bone pain. **Kanis** noted that the diphosphonates, the calcitonins and mithramycin are capable of inducing marked suppression of disease activity for prolonged periods. Whereas the effects of the calcitonins and mithramycin persist only for the duration of treatment, diphosphonate treatment consistently results in a reduction of disease activity for many months after stopping treatment. Current indications for long term treatment are debated. A major disadvantage of calcitonin is that it must normally be given by injection.

Radiology

Maldague B, Malghem J **Dynamic radiologic patterns of Paget's disease of bone** Clin Orthop 1987;217:126–151

Maldague studied sequential radiographs of 19 untreated patients followed for 6 years. Progressive extension of the lesions along the involved bone is one of the major characteristics of the disease. The mode of spread with remodelling of early and late disease is discussed. Examples of the sequential stages of the disease with types of resorption are illustrated.

Sarcoma

Schajowicz F, Araujo ES, Berenstein M **Sarcoma complicating Paget's disease of bone: a clinicopathological study of 62 cases** J Bone Joint Surg [Br] 1983;65B:299–307

Schajowicz reviewed the clinical and pathological features of 62 cases of sarcomatous change in Paget's disease. Most of the sarcomas occurred in polyostotic disease. Tumours often develop simultaneously, or at short time intervals, in the same or different bones. The histological features are characteristic. The prognosis is poor and survival after 5 years is very rare.

Hip Arthroplasty

MacDonald DJ, Sim FH **Total hip arthroplasty in Paget's disease – a follow-up note** J Bone Joint Surg [Am] 1987;69A:766–772

MacDonald discussed experience with total arthroplasty in 91 hips. The results were compared with a similar study of patients with no evidence of Paget's disease. There was an increased rate of revision for aseptic loosening in patients with Paget's disease. However, the overall results were good or excellent in 74%, suggesting that replacement of the hip using cemented components remains an acceptable form of treatment.

Lumbar Stenosis

Weisz GM **Lumbar canal stenosis in Paget's disease: the staging of the clinical syndrome, its diagnosis and treatment** Clin Orthop 1986;206:223–227

Weisz has drawn attention to the stages of development of stenosis of the lumbar canal in Paget's disease based on a study of 12 cases. The treatment for Stage I (early) is a short course of calcitonin for symptomatic relief. In the third stage, with radiculopathy, a decompression is necessary.

Osteopetrosis

Kaplan FS, August CS, Fallon MD, Dalinka M, Axel L, Haddad JG **Successful treatment of infantile malignant osteopetrosis by bone marrow transplantation: a case report** J Bone Joint Surg [Am] 1988;70A:617–623

Infantile malignant osteopetrosis (Albers–Schoenberg), or marble bone disease, is thought to result from congenital failure of osteoclastic bone resorption. Walker has demonstrated that this condition can be reversed by bone marrow transplantation. **Kaplan** has reported a case in detail with a 5-year follow-up. Studies of osteopetrosis provide opportunities to investigate the cell biology of the osteoclast and remodelling of bone.

Neuromuscular Disorders

Cerebral Palsy

The assessment and management of patients with cerebral palsy is both highly specialised and complicated. The authors have therefore chosen review chapters or articles which provide a rapid lead-in to principles rather than papers which concentrate on specific topics.

General Review

Rang M, Silver R, De La Garza J **Cerebral palsy** In: Lovell WW, Winter RB, eds. Paediatric orthopaedics. 2nd edn. Philadelphia: J B Lippincott Co, 1986: 345–396

Rang provided a general review of the subject. The differential diagnosis, examination for planning treatment and management were discussed. Rules were debated which should be observed before operation; there are many anecdotal figures which emphasise principles and lighten the text. Problems were described that can be encountered in different parts of the body. The management was classified into those who will never walk, the diplegic and the hemiplegic. A number of valuable aphorisms are included to guide treatment.

The Upper Limb

Skoff H, Woodbury D **Current concepts review: management of the upper extremity in cerebral palsy** J Bone Joint Surg [Am] 1985;67A:500–503

Fulford GE **The upper limb in cerebral palsy** In: Lamb DW, Hooper G, Kuczynski K, eds. The practice of hand surgery. 2nd edn. Oxford: Blackwell Scientific Publications, 1989:455–465

Skoff stressed the general approach to management of the upper extremity. The rare surgical candidate is an intelligent, well-motivated patient with spastic hemiplegia and demonstrable control of the limb. The best time for intervention is between the ages of 4 and 8 years. Details of technique were outlined; the most gratifying results were those of improvement in function of the hand in activities of daily living. **Fulford** classified problems by neurological presentation and stated that selected patients can be helped by surgery. A surgical programme must be organised according to the type and severity of the deformity. Spastic muscles cannot be used as transfers with the same effectiveness as muscles which are normal.

The Lower Limb

Hoffer MM **Current concepts review: management of the hip in cerebral palsy** J Bone Joint Surg [Am] 1986;68A:629–631

Gage JR **Surgical treatment of knee dysfunction in cerebral palsy** Clin Orthop 1990;253:45–54

Fulford GE **Surgical management of ankle and foot deformities in cerebral palsy** Clin Orthop 1990;253:55–61

Hoffer presented a short review of a complex dynamic problem. Controversies in treatment were considered in turn for a patient with overactive adductors, an unstable subluxated hip and a dislocated hip. When a deformity of the spine and a dislocated hip were both present, Hoffer considered that the spine should always be corrected first, since fixed pelvic obliquity maintains the dislocation of the hip. Many patients with spastic diplegia stop walking in adolescence; it is suggested that surgical procedures will prolong their ability to walk. **Gage** discussed normal knee joint mechanics and the gait in cerebral palsy. In the crouch gait, hamstring lengthening alone may convert a flexed-knee gait to an extended-knee stiff-legged gait. Restoration of normal knee function in patients with spastic paralysis is more successful with fractional hamstring lengthening combined with transfer of the rectus femoris tendon to the iliotibial band or the tendon of semitendinosis. Fulford described a system of surgical treatment of deformities of the ankle and foot based on experience with 420 children. Types of deformity were classified into three groups – fixed, dynamic and mixed, each treated differently. The most common indication for foot surgery was equinus deformity. Tendo-achilles lengthening was satisfactory for fixed equinus and transfer of the medial belly and tendon of the gastrocnemius to the dorsum of the foot for dynamic equinus. The treatment of hindfoot valgus and varus was debated.

The Spine

Fergusson RL, Allen BL **Considerations in the treatment of cerebral palsy patients with spinal deformities** Orthop Clin North Am 1988;19:2:419–425

Rinsky LA **Surgery of spine deformity in cerebral palsy: 12 years in the evolution of scoliosis management** Clin Orthop 1990;253:100–109

Fergusson stressed the problems of deformity in cerebral palsy, which are different from those in idiopathic scoliosis. Progression of the deformity may occur after skeletal maturity. Significant pseudarthrosis may occur after fusion, especially when posterior arthrodesis is used as the sole procedure. The cerebral palsy patient is prone to regression after surgery. **Rinsky** discussed lessons learned from 12 years of surgery on patients with cerebral palsy and spinal deformity. Most patients were retarded non-walkers who had total body involvement, with pelvic obliquity and severe thoracolumbar curves. Three different techniques were employed. The general trend was towards longer fusion with a two-stage anterior discectomy and fusion followed by posterior fusion. Luque rod instrumentation without fusion has been abandoned.

Book Reference

Bleck EE **Orthopaedic management in cerebral palsy.** McKeith Press, Oxford: Blackwell Scientific Publications, 1987

The book published by **Bleck** is included here as the most useful authoritative source of reference on this large, complicated subject. There are chapters on goals, treatment and management (page 142), spastic hemiplegia (page 213) and spastic diplegia (page 282).

Stroke

Braun RM, West F, Mooney V, Nickel VL, Roper BA, Caldwell C **Surgical treatment of the painful shoulder contracture in the stroke patient** J Bone Joint Surg [Am] 1971;53A:1307–1312

Waters RL, Garland DE, Perry J, Habig T, Slabaugh P **Stiff-legged gait in hemiplegia: surgical correction** J Bone Joint Surg [Am] 1979;61A:927–933

Roper B **Rehabilitation after a stroke** J Bone Joint Surg [Br] 1982;64B: 156–163

Braun debated the value of surgical release and an immediate postoperative exercise regimen for patients who have had a stroke with a painful internal rotation contracture of the shoulder. **Waters** described an evaluation of 126 patients with unilateral stiff-legged gait following a stroke or other cerebral lesions. Selective tenotomy of the quadriceps may improve knee flexion and gait in some of these patients. **Roper** stressed the paramount importance of early mobilisation following a stroke. Surgery does have a part to play once a stable neurological state has been reached. However, results may be unpredictable. Loss of heel-strike is a major obstacle to effective gait. Correction of obstructive spasticity can be accomplished by surgical release of appropriate tendons and by selective neurectomy. The use of various operations in the arm and leg are discussed.

Spina Bifida

There has been a marked reduction in the incidence of myelomeningocele in the last decade due, in part, to improved antenatal diagnosis and selective abortion. The authors have therefore chosen references which are largely recent and reflect current topics of debate.

Review Articles

Sharrard WJW **The orthopaedic management of spina bifida – general considerations** In: Galasko CSB, ed. Neuromuscular problems in orthopaedics. Oxford: Blackwell Scientific Publications, 1987:45–56

Carroll NC **Assessment and management of the lower extremity in myelodysplasia** Orthop Clin North Am 1987;18:4:709–724

Asher M, Olson J **Factors affecting the ambulatory status of patients with spina bifida cystica** J Bone Joint Surg [Am] 1983;65A:350–356

McCarthy GT **Treating children with spina bifida: an individual programme for each child** Br Med J 1991;302:65–66

Sharrard provided an overview of the subject with discussion of the forms of meningocele, the nature and prognosis of the paralysis, the types of deformity, and both early and late orthopaedic management. **Carroll** discussed and illustrated motor function at different levels of paralysis. Common knee deformities seen are recurvatum, flexion contracture and valgus. The goal in managing deformities of the foot is to achieve a plantigrade posture with stable skin. **Asher** studied factors affecting ambulation in 98 patients. The most important variable is the neurosegmental level of paraplegia. Patients with third lumbar and higher levels of paraplegia usually become non-ambulatory, whereas patients with fourth lumbar or lower levels remain functional walkers. Prevention of obesity and musculoskeletal deformity is important to maintain ambulation. **McCarthy** reviewed the controversies in early treatment of babies with myelomeningocele and provided a rapid update on the paediatric approach to their management.

The Hip

Carroll NC, Sharrard WJW **Long-term follow-up of posterior iliopsoas transplantation for paralytic dislocation of the hip** J Bone Joint Surg [Am] 1972;54A:551–560

Drummond DS, Moreau M, Cruess RL **The results and complications of surgery for the paralytic hip and spine in myelomeningocele** J Bone Joint Surg [Br] 1980;62B:49–53

Stillwell A, Menelaus MB **Walking ability after transplantation of the iliopsoas: a long-term follow-up** J Bone Joint Surg [Br] 1984;66B:656–659

Weisl H, Fairclough JA, Jones DG **Stabilisation of the hip in myelo-meningocele: comparison of posterior iliopsoas transfer and varus rotation osteotomy** J Bone Joint Surg [Br] 1988;70B:29–33

The management of the hip in spina bifida is controversial. **Carroll** studied the natural history of hip instability with various neurosegmental levels of paralysis. Muscle imbalance is an important cause of instability. In 58 hips the operative treatment included a posterior iliopsoas transplant. Review 5–10 years later showed that although hip stability was achieved in many patients, instability was still present in 40%. Many of these children were capable of some form of independent gait. **Drummond** reviewed the results of operations to stabilise the deformed spine or unstable hip in 40 patients. Stabilisation of the hip was achieved in 69% but improved walking in only 27%. It was concluded that posterior transfer alone will not stabilise a hip which is already dysplastic, and seldom improves walking. **Stillwell** discussed results in 47 patients with transplantation of the iliopsoas performed more than 10 years previously. The walking ability was not jeopardised by the loss of hip flexor power, but the power of the transfer was poor. The operation should not be performed within the first year of life and it should only be carried out in those patients likely to walk in below-knee splints, and who will be able to continue walking in adult life. **Weisl** compared the results of iliopsoas transfer and varus rotation osteotomy. The technical results of both operations were satisfactory. The varus rotation osteotomy with psoas division, adductor tenotomy and anterior obturator neurectomy was at least as effective in stabilising the hip as an iliopsoas transfer.

The Foot

Malhotra D, Puri R, Owen R **Valgus deformity of the ankle in children with spina bifida aperta** J Bone Joint Surg [Br] 1984;66B:381–385

Olney BW, Menelaus MB **Triple arthrodesis of the foot in spina bifida patients** J Bone Joint Surg [Br] 1988;70B:234–235

Lang-Stevenson AI, Sharrard WJW, Betts RP, Duckworth T **Neuropathic ulcers of the foot** J Bone Joint Surg [Br] 1985;67B:438–442

Malhotra studied 35 ankles with a valgus deformity of the hindfoot in 23 children. He noted that the ankle is often the main site of the deformity. It was concluded that operations performed below the ankle are unlikely to succeed and that the deformity needs to be corrected above the ankle by epiphysiodesis or supramalleolar osteotomy. **Olney** reviewed the results of triple arthrodesis at an average of 10 years after operation. The operation is demanding, but once the deformity is corrected and a solid fusion obtained, the results do not deteriorate with time. It is a reliable procedure for achieving a stable foot. **Lang-Stevenson** reported a prospective study of the causes and treatment of 26 long-standing neuropathic ulcers of the foot. Prevention of deformity is the best means of avoiding these ulcers. The treatment of choice for an established ulcer, however large, is the application of serial skin-tight plaster casts with relief from weight bearing. Healing of the ulcer is only the preliminary treatment; the cause must then be defined and corrected if recurrence is to be prevented.

Orthotic Treatment

Rose GK, Sankarankutty M, Stallard J **The clinical review of the orthotic treatment of myelomeningocele patients** J Bone Joint Surg [Br] 1983;65B: 242–246

Rose analysed 100 patients with a myelomeningocele. The use of the "swivel walker" and "hip guidance orthosis" has been associated with an improved level of function. Over 30% of patients with thoracic lesions and 68% of those with lumbar lesions achieved independent walking.

Book Reference

Menelaus MB **The orthopaedic management of spina bifida cystica.** 2nd edn. Edinburgh: Churchill Livingstone, 1980

The detailed monograph by **Menelaus** contains much further information on this large subject, including especially orthoses (pages 67–76) and the management of spinal problems (pages 152–187).

Poliomyelitis

With the advent of immunisation, poliomyelitis is no longer a problem in the Western world and recent references in the literature are rare. On the other hand, the disease is still common in the Middle and Far East and many developing countries.

The Classic

Sharrard WJW **The distribution of the permanent paralysis in the lower limb in poliomyelitis: a clinical and pathological study** J Bone Joint Surg [Br] 1955;37B:540–558

Sharrard analysed the distribution of the permanent paresis and paralysis in the muscles of 203 lower limbs affected by poliomyelitis, and this was related to the destruction of motor nerve cells in the spinal cord. Some muscles, for example tibialis anterior, are more often paralysed than paretic because they are innervated by short motor columns. Muscles such as the hip flexors are more often paretic than paralysed and these are innervated by long columns. There are characteristic patterns of muscle paralysis which result in the lower limb.

Clinical Study

Kumar K, Kapahtia NK **The pattern of muscle involvement in poliomyelitis of the upper limb** Int Orthop 1986;10:11–15

Kumar studied the pattern of muscle paralysis in the upper limb in 31 children in India. The most frequently paralysed muscle was the deltoid. The next most commonly affected were the elbow flexors and extensors.

Surgical Treatment

Brooks D **Surgery for poliomyelitis** Curr Orthop 1989;3:101–105

James JIP **Poliomyelitis: essentials of surgical management.** London: Edward Arnold, 1987

Ingram AJ **Poliomyelitis** In: Crenshaw AH, ed. Campbell's operative orthopaedics. 7th edn. St Louis, Washington DC, Toronto: CV Mosby & Co, 1987:2926–3022

Brooks provided a short review of the indications for and general principles of surgical treatment, including the management of contractures, tendon transfers to restore muscle imbalance, correction of limb shortening and stabilisation. A concise account was produced by **James** to guide the surgeon trying to manage the effects of this disease with little or no relevant experience. **Ingram** debated treatment in detail, with a description of the many operative procedures that were commonly used in the past.

Arthrogryposis Multiplex Congenita

Clinical Studies

Shapiro F, Bresnan MJ **Current concepts review: orthopaedic management of childhood neuromuscular disease. II. peripheral neuropathies Friedreich's ataxia and arthrogryposis multiplex congenita** J Bone Joint Surg [Am] 1982; 64A:951–953

Lloyd-Roberts GC, Lettin AWF **Arthrogryposis multiplex congenita** J Bone Joint Surg [Br] 1970;52B:497–507

Staheli LT, Chew DE, Elliot JS, Mosca VS **Management of hip dislocations in children with arthrogryposis** J Pediatr Orthop 1987;7:681–685

Green ADL, Fixsen JA, Lloyd-Roberts GC **Talectomy for arthrogryposis multiplex congenita** J Bone Joint Surg [Br] 1984;66B:697–699

Williams PF **Management of upper limb problems in arthrogryposis** Clin Orthop 1985;194:60–67

Shapiro summarised arthrogryposis, stressing the need for accurate diagnosis and assessment. In the lower limb, multiple operations are often required. They should commence early and be followed by a prolonged period of splintage to prevent recurrent deformity. The upper limb is more resistant to effective surgical treatment. Function may be adequate even in the presence of severe deformity. **Lloyd-Roberts** detailed 39 patients and discussed both the general principles of management and the specific surgical options for various joint deformities. **Staheli** recommended reduction of the dislocated hip to prevent the development of pelvic obliquity and scoliosis. He favoured the medial approach to avoid capsulorrhaphy, which restricts joint movement. **Green** emphasised the importance of a plantigrade foot. Talectomy was performed in 34 feet in which conservative management and soft-tissue surgery had failed. At late review, 71% were plantigrade. In a symposium on the problems associated with arthrogryposis **Williams** discussed the management of upper limb deformities emphasising the evaluation of disability rather than deformity. Surgery is indicated particularly at the elbow to obtain mobility. Wrist arthrodesis and derotation osteotomy of the humerus may also be necessary.

Other Neuromuscular Disorders

Shapiro F, Bresnan MJ **Current concepts review: orthopaedic management of childhood neuromuscular disease. I. Spinal muscular atrophy** J Bone Joint Surg [Am] 1982;64A:785–789

Shapiro F, Bresnan MJ **Current concepts review: orthopaedic management of childhood neuromuscular disease. II. Peripheral neuropathies, Friedreich's ataxia and arthrogryposis multiplex congenita** J Bone Joint Surg [Am] 1982;64A:949–951

Shapiro F, Bresnan MJ **Current concepts review: orthopaedic management of childhood neuromuscular disease. III. Diseases of muscle** J Bone Joint Surg [Am] 1982;64A:1102–1107

Three papers have been included which provide information on rare neuromuscular problems which may require orthopaedic management. In Part I, **Shapiro** described the characteristics of infantile and juvenile spinal atrophy. These patients present with widespread weakness and the majority are never able to walk. Part II discusses the characteristics of peroneal muscular atrophy, usually inherited and presenting with a high-stepping gait, wasting and progressive pes cavus. In Part III **Shapiro** summarised knowledge and the orthopaedic management of patients with Duchenne muscular dystrophy. Patients rarely survive beyond the late teens. The disease only involves males and demonstrates recessive inheritance. The management of scoliosis is discussed elsewhere (page 106).

Rheumatoid Disorders

In this section, the authors have been conscious of the increasing growth of rheumatology and the need of orthopaedic surgeons for basic knowledge of the rheumatic diseases.

Rheumatoid Arthritis

Pathology

Helliwell TR Surgical pathology of rheumatoid disease In: Beddow FH, ed. The surgical management of rheumatoid arthritis. London: Wright, 1988:19–36

Gardner DL **The pathology of rheumatoid arthritis** In: Scott JT, ed. Copeman's textbook of the rheumatic diseases. 6th edn, Vol I. Edinburgh: Churchill Livingstone, 1986:604–652

Helliwell discussed articular pathology including pannus, changes in the cartilage and para-articular tissues. The systemic effects of the disease are outlined. Generalised osteoporosis may affect about 25% of patients. The most severe type of disease includes necrotising arthritis. Muscle weakness and wasting are common features. **Gardner** provided a comprehensive reference chapter to this subject. There is increased risk of infection, especially with anaerobic organisms. For each sex at each year of follow-up, the cumulative survival rate in rheumatoid arthritis is lower than normal.

Radiology

Watt I **Imaging for rheumatoid arthritis** Curr Orthop 1989;3:141–145

Watt discussed imaging and its value in establishing the diagnosis and activity of the disease. The value of MRI is outstanding in defining granulation tissue around the odontoid peg and atlantoaxial instability.

Prognosis

Fleming A, Crown JM, Corbett M **Prognostic value of early features in rheumatoid disease** Br Med J 1976;1:1243–1245

Fleming described the outcome of 102 patients who presented within a year of onset and were observed for 5 years. One quarter were improved but 60% had a severe or deteriorating condition. Factors which adversely affected prognosis included older age at onset, underweight, many affected joints and involvement of the wrist or metatarsophalangeal joints.

Treatment

Corbett M **The management of rheumatoid disease** In: Scott JT, ed. Copeman's textbook of the rheumatic diseases. 6th edn, Vol I. Edinburgh: Churchill Livingstone, 1986:706–719

Pullar T, Wright V **Current drug treatment of rheumatoid arthritis** Curr Orthop 1988;2:247–253

Wright V **The treatment of severe rheumatoid arthritis** Br Med J 1986;292: 431–432

Corbett discussed management. The worst problem for the patient is fear: he is frightened of losing independence and becoming a burden to others. Medication and drugs are debated. The extra-articular complications and their management are described, including those involving the cardiovascular system, the lungs, neuropathies and the eyes. Any operation, however dramatic, is only one incident in the total management of the patient. **Pullar** presented an outline of the drug treatment of rheumatoid arthritis. The simple analgesic of choice is paracetamol. The non-steroidal anti-inflammatory drugs are classified and their use debated. Aspirin is the most commonly used salicylate and in high doses is effective, although gastrointestinal toxicity may be a problem. The value of second-line drugs including intramuscular gold and penicillamine is described. Most antirheumatoid drugs display significant toxicity. **Wright** reviewed management of the patient with intractable destructive rheumatoid arthritis. Drastic measures may be necessary such as the use of azathioprine or methotrexate; such treatment is the realm of the expert physician.

Surgery

Mowat AG **The surgical treatment of arthritis** In: Scott JT, ed. Copeman's textbook of the rheumatic diseases. 6th edn, Vol II. Edinburgh: Churchill Livingstone, 1986:1518–1565

Mowat discussed general surgical considerations in the treatment of arthritis. Factors which influence wound healing, drug therapy and thromboembolism and its prevention are debated. (This paper has been included at this stage as an introduction to the detailed references presented elsewhere.)

Book Reference

Scott JT ed. **Copeman's textbook of the rheumatic diseases**. 6th edn, Vols I and II. Edinburgh: Churchill Livingstone, 1986

This book has excellent chapters on other aspects of the rheumatoid diseases and is included for reference.

Seronegative Spondarthritis

Moll JMH, Haslock I, Wright V **The seronegative spondarthritides** In: Scott JT, ed. Copeman's textbook of the rheumatic diseases. 6th edn, Vol I. Edinburgh: Churchill Livingstone, 1986:723–744

Burns TM, Calin A **Hand radiograph as a diagnostic discriminant between the "seropositive" and "seronegative" rheumatoid arthritis: a controlled study** Ann Rheum Dis 1983;42:605–612

Moll reviewed the concept of seronegative arthritis and the diseases it includes. The idea represents the most recent milestone in the evolution of rheumatological nomenclature. Criteria are described, including absence of rheumatoid factor and subcutaneous nodules but presence of radiological sacroiliitis and peripheral arthritis. Conditions such as ankylosing spondylitis, psoriatic arthritis and Reiter's disease are included. There is some "overlap" between members of the group. These disorders are not variants of rheumatoid arthritis and an optimistic prognosis can be given to the patient. **Burns** suggested that the radiographs of the hands of patients with seronegative disease have distinctive characteristics compared with those who are seropositive. There is a relative absence of subchondral erosions, more new bone formation and more asymmetrical involvement.

Psoriatic Arthritis

Wright V **Psoriatic arthritis** In: Scott JT, ed. Copeman's textbook of the rheumatic diseases. 6th edn, Vol I. Edinburgh: Churchill Livingstone, 1986: 775–786

Wright noted that there was increasing clinical, radiographic and serological evidence to support the classification of psoriatic arthritis as a true entity; it is present in a small percentage of patients with psoriasis. Clinical features are debated and various types recognised. This type of arthritis produces less pain and disability than rheumatoid arthritis.

Ankylosing Spondylitis

Review Article

Bossingham DH, Dickson RA, In: Dickson RA, ed. **Spinal surgery: science and practice.** London: Butterworths, 1990:216–232

Bossingham and **Dickson** provided a recent review of the pathology, presentation, complications and treatment, both medical and surgical, of ankylosing spondylitis. The most widely used drugs in the United Kingdom are probably indomethacin, naproxen and ibuprofen, all of which have been demonstrated to be effective in comparison with placebo in double-blind studies. The orthopaedic aspects of this disease are narrated, including the complications of fractures of the spine and kyphosis.

Natural History

Carette S, Graham D, Little H, Rubenstein J, Rosen P **The natural disease course of ankylosing spondylitis** Arthritis Rheum 1983;26:2:186–190

Carette discussed the natural history of the disease based on a study of a large number of war veterans for many years. After 38 years, 92% of the patients were functioning well and only 40% had progressed to severe spinal restriction. A predictable pattern of disease emerged within the first 10 years. If hip disease has not developed within the first 10 years, it is unlikely to do so.

The Hip

Bisla RS, Ranawat CS, Inglis AE **Total hip replacement in patients with ankylosing spondylitis with involvement of the hip** J Bone Joint Surg [Am] 1976;58A:233–238

Williams E, Taylor AR, Arden GP, Edwards DH **Arthroplasty of the hip in ankylosing spondylitis** J Bone Joint Surg [Br] 1977;59B:393–397

Bisla described good results in a high percentage of 34 total hip arthroplasties observed for 3.5 years. Particular benefit occurred in posture and function, resulting in gainful employment. Most of the limited motion in ankylosing spondylitis was due to myositis ossificans. **Williams** obtained 73% good or excellent results up to 10 years after total hip arthroplasty. Complications included deep infection, but the most troublesome problem was recurrence of ankylosis, both bony and fibrous.

The Spine

McMaster MJ **A technique for lumbar spinal osteotomy in ankylosing spondylitis** J Bone Joint Surg [Br] 1985;67B:204–210

McMaster discussed experience of 14 patients with ankylosing spondylitis who had an extension osteotomy for severe flexion deformity of the spine. The Smith–Peterson technique was modified, which allowed a slow, controlled closure of the osteotomy followed by rigid fixation, and no serious complications occurred. Assessment of the deformity and technique of surgery was described and this was related to the previous contributions of Adams (1952) and Law (1959). The paper is a useful reference for this rare but difficult problem.

Book Reference

Moll JMH **Ankylosing spondylitis** In: Scott JT, ed. Copeman's textbook of the rheumatic diseases. 6th edn, Vol I. Edinburgh: Churchill Livingstone, 1986: 745–774

Moll produced a reference chapter on ankylosing spondylitis, including the more recent developments in knowledge of aetiology, pathology and management.

Chronic Juvenile Arthritis

Clinical Studies

Ansell BM, Swann M **Review article: the management of chronic arthritis of children** J Bone Joint Surg [Br] 1983;65B:536–543

Swann M, Ansell BM **Soft-tissue release, of the hips in children with juvenile chronic arthritis** J Bone Joint Surg [Br] 1986;68B:404–408

Ruddlesdin C, Ansell BM, Arden GP, Swann M **Total hip replacement in children with juvenile chronic arthritis** J Bone Joint Surg [Br] 1986;68B: 218–222

Sarokhan AJ, Scott RD, Thomas WH, Sledge CB, Ewald FC, Cloos DW **Total knee arthroplasty in juvenile rheumatoid arthritis** J Bone Joint Surg [Am] 1983;65A:1071–1080

From her unique experience, **Ansell** provided a comprehensive review of both the medical and surgical management of chronic arthritis in children. Surgical procedures include soft-tissue release, synovectomy, stapling and total replacement. **Swann** reported the use of 89 tenotomies for flexion and adduction deformities around the hip. These proved a safe and effective method of relieving pain and improving function. More extensive soft-tissue release operations offered no advantage and recovery was often more painful and prolonged. The results of 75 total hip replacements were reported by **Ruddlesdin** with a mean follow-up of 5 years. Careful selection is essential and the results obtained were gratifying. Constant assessment by a rheumatologist is essential. **Sarokhan** reported the follow-up of 29 knee replacements after an average of 5 years. All but one patient became a limited or full community walker. Custom-made components were often required. Skeletal immaturity was not an absolute contraindication to surgery. Marked improvement in knee function and quality of life made the short- and long-term risk of knee implant surgery worth while.

Reiter's Disease

Wright V **Reiter's disease** In: Scott JT, ed. Copeman's textbook of the rheumatic diseases. 6th edn, Vol I. Edinburgh: Churchill Livingstone, 1986:787–801

Wright produced a useful article which provides update knowledge on this condition with particular reference to its clinical features and associated urogenital lesions. Periostitis may be a striking feature, including both the hands and the feet with plantar spurs.

Gout and Degenerative Osteoarthritis

Gout

Dieppe P, Calvert P **Gout** In: Crystals and joint disease. London: Chapman & Hall, 1983:115–153, 248–250

Gout is essentially a medical condition but is occasionally encountered by the orthopaedic surgeon. One reference has therefore been provided. **Dieppe** and **Calvert** have produced a useful reference chapter which discusses the epidemiology, pathology, clinical aspects and treatment of acute and chronic gout.

Pyrophosphate Arthropathy (Pseudogout: Chondrocalcinosis)

Dieppe P, Calvert P **Calcium pyrophosphate dihydrate deposition** In: Crystals and joint disease. London: Chapman & Hall, 1983: 154–188

In the past 20 years there has been an increase in awareness of the frequency of calcium deposition in pathological joints. **Dieppe** and **Calvert** discussed in detail chondrocalcinosis (otherwise called pseudogout), its diagnosis and treatment. Although usually idiopathic, it may be associated with other diseases such as hyperparathyroidism, haemochromatosis or diabetes. Its presentation as an acute arthritis in 105 patients is discussed. The diagnosis is confirmed by finding the characteristic birefringement crystals in the synovial fluid. The features of chronic arthritis in association with pyrophosphate deposition are discussed with illustrative X-rays (pages 180–183). Deposits may be asymptomatic or they can occur in association with chronic destructive changes. The treatment of chronic pyrophosphate arthropathy is debated.

Osteoarthritis

The Classic

Harrison MHM, Schajowicz F, Truetta J **Osteoarthritis of the hip: a study of the nature and evolution of the disease** J Bone Joint Surg [Br] 1953;35B: 598–626

The study by **Harrison** was based on an analysis of 91 postmortem examinations of the hip, 45 femoral heads removed at operation for osteoarthritis and radiographs from 80 patients followed over several years. Daily use was found to preserve rather than "wear out" articular cartilage; the vigorous attempt at repair after degeneration was thought to increase vascularity, so weakening bone and leading to collapse.

Pathology

Freeman MAR **Pathogenesis of osteoarthritis: a hypothesis** Ann Rheum Dis 1975;34: Suppl;120–121

Radin EL, Paul IL, Rose RM **Role of mechanical factors in pathogenesis of primary osteoarthritis** Lancet 1972;1:519–522

Kempson GE **Mechanical properties of articular cartilage and their relationship to matrix degradation and age** Ann Rheum Dis 1975;34:Suppl;111–113

Jeffery AK **Osteogenesis in the osteoarthritic femoral head: a study using radioactive ^{32}P and tetracycline bone markers** J Bone Joint Surg [Br] 1973; 55B:262–272

Jeffery AK **Osteophytes and the osteoarthritic femoral head** J Bone Joint Surg [Br] 1975;57B:314–324

Bullough PG **The pathology of degenerative change in the hip: the microscopic changes** In: Reynolds D, Freeman M, eds. Osteoarthritis in the young adult hip. Edinburgh: Churchill Livingstone, 1989:36–49

Freeman M **The pathology of degenerative change in the hip: gross changes and their surgical implications** In: Reynolds D, Freeman M, eds. Osteoarthritis in the young adult hip. Edinburgh: Churchill Livingstone, 1989:49–57

Freeman, in a symposium on pathogenesis, suggested that osteoarthrosis is the non-specific end result of a number of pathological processes and could be viewed as "joint failure" (analogous to heart failure). Surface defects in articular cartilage added to repetitive high contact force may lead to fatigue failure in the collagen network. **Kempson** showed a decrease in strength of the surface layers of articular cartilage which is associated with alterations in matrix composition. This suggested a mechanical defect in the collagen network. **Radin** suggested that joints wear out by repetitive impulsive loading, rather than by rubbing. Many examples of the epidemiology of osteoarthrosis, as well as the pattern of joint involvement, were quoted in support of this hypothesis. **Jeffery** noted that remodelling of bone structure is a distinctive feature of osteoarthritis, particularly in its more advanced stages. He analysed osteogenesis in the osteoarthritic femoral head with radioactive ^{32}P and tetracycline bone markers. In advanced osteoarthritis, considerable osteogenic activity was observed in either enchondral ossification or apposition of new bone to existing trabeculae. In a further paper (1975) **Jeffery** studied the morphology and growth of osteophytes in 40 femoral heads removed from patients with advanced osteoarthritis. The pattern of osteophyte formation appeared to be influenced by the direction and degree of displacement of the femoral head in relation to the acetabulum.

Aetiology and Patterns

Solomon L **Patterns of osteoarthritis of the hip** J Bone Joint Surg [Br] 1976; 58B:176–183

Harris WH **Etiology of osteoarthritis of the hip** Clin Orthop 1986;213:20–33

Huskisson EC, Dieppe PA, Tucker AK, Cannell LB **Another look at osteo-arthritis** Ann Rheum Dis 1979;38:423–428

Dieppe PA, Doherty M, MacFarlane DG, Hutton CW, Bradfield JW, Watt I **Apatite-associated destructive arthritis** Br J Rheum 1984;23:84–91

Solomon questioned the traditional concept of division of osteoarthritis into primary – an intrinsic defect of cartilage – and secondary resulting from previous articular damage. The hypothesis was advanced that osteoarthritis is always secondary to some underlying abnormality of the joint and this was supported by a detailed analysis of 327 cases of osteoarthritis of the hip. Some predisposing abnormality of the joint was usually diagnosed, including Perthes' disease, epiphysiolysis, acetabular dysplasia and features suggesting an underlying inflammatory arthritis. **Harris** agreed with Solomon and stated that 90% of patients with so-called primary osteoarthritis of the hips, when adequately assessed, showed abnormalities in the hip joint, the most common being mild acetabular dysplasia or a pistol-grip deformity. He considered that primary osteoarthritis of the hip is rare or non-existent. **Huskisson** reviewed 100 consecutive cases of osteoarthritis seen in a medical clinic and contrasted these with 100 patients with rheumatoid disease. Osteoarthritis was usually a polyarticular disease and evidence of inflammation was often found, including morning stiffness, redness of distal interphalangeal joints and effusions in the knees. He suggested that these findings do not support the concept of osteoarthritis as a mechanical non-inflammatory wear-and-tear condition, and a primary abnormality of articular cartilage was suggested. **Dieppe** described 12 patients with a distinctive type of destructive arthropathy. The principle joints affected were the shoulder and knee. In some, extensive calcific material was seen in the synovium and most patients had some associated joint disorder. The aetiological role of crystals in the joint was discussed.

Osteoarthritis and Osteoporosis

Dequeker J The relationship between osteoporosis and osteoarthritis Clin Rheum Dis 1985;11:271–291

Dequeker compared postmenopausal osteoporotic and osteoarthritic cases and found that they represent two different populations: first, osteoporosis with slender body status and few degenerative joint changes, and second, osteoarthritis with above normal bone mass, more muscle strength and fewer fractures. Cases with clinical osteoporosis have a rate of bone loss greater than normal, whereas primary osteoarthritic cases have a slower bone loss with age. The results of oestrogen and growth hormone treatment are considered. Data are presented which support the concept that postmenopausal osteoporosis and osteoarthritis are two different disease entities and not simply the end result of normal ageing, aggravated by wear-and-tear phenomena.

Haemophilic Arthropathy

Pathology

Stein H, Duthie RB The pathogenesis of chronic haemophilic arthropathy J Bone Joint Surg [Br] 1981;63B:601–609

Clinical Studies

Aronstam A, Browne RS, Wassef M, Hamad Z The clinical features of early bleeding into the muscles of the lower limb in severe haemophiliacs J Bone Joint Surg [Br] 1983;65B:19–23

Railton GT, Aronstam A **Early bleeding into upper limb muscles in severe haemophilia: clinical features and treatment** J Bone Joint Surg [Br] 1987;69B: 100–102

Wilson DJ, McLardy-Smith PD, Woodham CH, MacLarnon JC **Diagnostic ultrasound in haemophilia** J Bone Joint Surg [Br] 1987;69B:103–107

Atkins RM, Henderson NJ, Duthie RB **Joint contractures in the hemophilias** Clin Orthop 1987;219:97–106

Stein summarised basic knowledge of the pathology of haemophilia and studied specimens of tissue from synovium and articular cartilage collected from 39 patients. The synovium becomes progressively fibrotic and the hyaline cartilage degenerates. Enzymatic processes appear to be responsible for the degradation of the articular cartilage. **Aronstam** described the clinical features and management of 178 early bleeding episodes in the lower limb. Eighty per cent of bleeding in muscle in haemophiliacs occurs in the quadriceps and calf muscles. The first symptom was often pain on movement. Ninety-five per cent of all bleeds were treated in less than 3 hours from onset of symptoms. **Railton** and **Aronstam** later described the features of early bleeding in the upper limb in 44 patients. The most frequent site was the deltoid muscle. A policy of early treatment was effective in prompting rapid complete recovery. **Wilson** discussed the value of ultrasound in the diagnosis of bleeding in haemophilia. The technique was outlined and the characteristics and significance of the echo pattern discussed. Ultrasound may considerably assist the management of these cases. The pathology and treatment of joint contractures was debated by **Atkins**. Contracture was seen most commonly as an equinus at the ankle, or flexion at the knee or elbow. The cause is either fibrosis following intramuscular haematoma or chronic changes in the joint following recurrent haemarthroses. The introduction of home therapy is an important preventive measure.

Arthrodesis or Arthroplasty?

Houghton GR, Dickson RA **Lower limb arthrodeses in haemophilia** J Bone Joint Surg [Br] 1978;60B:387–389

Lachiewicz PF, Inglis AE, Insall JN, Sculco TP, Hilgartner MW, Bussel JB **Total knee arthroplasty in haemophilia** J Bone Joint Surg [Am] 1985;67A: 1361–1366

Karthaus RP, Novakova IRO **Total knee replacement in haemophilic arthropathy** J Bone Joint Surg [Br] 1988;70B:382–385

Review Article

Luck JV, Kasper CK **Surgical management of advanced hemophilic arthropathy: an overview of 20 years' experience** Clin Orthop 1989;242:60–82

The management of the painful destroyed joint is controversial and never easy. **Houghton** in 1978 described the experience and results in 16 patients who had undergone arthrodesis of one joint in the lower limb. Two recent papers on knee arthroplasty are included in view of the interest in this subject. **Lachiewicz** obtained 21 good or excellent results in 24 knee arthroplasties, although with a short follow-up. The operation should be performed only with strict haematological supervision and the surgeon should be prepared to treat many potential complications. **Karthaus** on an experience of 11 total knee replacements stressed the high incidence of complications, but nevertheless, all patients were free of pain and all but one returned to employment. **Luck** has recently reviewed experience with 168 surgical procedures over 20 years. The paper discussed problems of the shoulder, elbow and hip as well as those of the knee and ankle. The aim was to determine appropriate indications for surgery and which procedures are most successful.

Bone Necrosis

Review Article

Solomon L **Avascular necrosis of bone**. In: Catterall A, ed. Recent advances in orthopaedics 5. Edinburgh: Churchill Livingstone,1987:43–60

Solomon provided an overview of the subject. The aetiology, pathogenesis and clinical features are debated and illustrated. Four stages are described from pre-clinical with no radiographic abnormality (Stage I), to the most advanced, characterised by articular destruction (Stage IV). The value of various treatment modalities is discussed, including medullary decompression, bone grafting, osteotomy, electrical stimulation and arthroplasty. A guide to management is given, depending upon the stage of the osteonecrosis.

Pathogenesis

Catto M A **Histological study of avascular necrosis of the femoral head after transcervical fracture** J Bone Joint Surg [Br] 1965;47B:749–776

Solomon L **Drug-induced arthropathy and necrosis of the femoral head** J Bone Joint Surg [Br] 1973;55B:246–261

Kenzora JE, Glimcher MJ **Pathogenesis of idiopathic osteonecrosis: the ubiquitous crescent sign** Orthop Clin North Am 1985;16:681–696

Saito S, Inoue A, Ono K **Intramedullary haemorrhage as a possible cause of avascular necrosis of the femoral head: the histology of 16 femoral heads at the silent stage** J Bone Joint Surg [Br] 1987;69B:346–351

Catto described the histological appearances of avascular necrosis after a fracture. This paper was included in the *Selected References in Orthopaedic Trauma* (1989 page 82) but is noted here for comparison with other types of osteonecrosis. **Solomon** described the common pathological lesion of "drug-induced arthropathy" which may follow corticosteroid therapy, alcoholism or analgesic abuse. The characteristic change is subchondral fragmentation and osteonecrosis followed by reactive bone formation and a typical increased radiographic density. **Kenzora** discussed osteonecrosis involving the head of the femur and also the distal femoral condyle, the proximal humerus and the talus. The natural history in various joints is described. The pathogenesis of the radiographic "crescent sign" is debated. The subchondral fracture which the sign represents is routinely found during repair. **Saito** studied core biopsy specimens from 16 femoral heads affected by idiopathic necrosis at the silent stage without clinical or radiographic manifestations. All showed haemorrhage associated with necrosis. It was concluded that repeated intramedullary haemorrhage at the silent stage is probably related to the pathogenesis of necrosis.

Treatment

Ficat RP **Review article: idiopathic bone necrosis of the femoral head: early diagnosis and treatment** J Bone Joint Surg [Br] 1985;67B:3–9

Meyers MH **Osteonecrosis of the femoral head treated with the muscle pedicle graft** Orthop Clin North Am 1985;16:741–745

Cornell CN, Salvati EA, Pellicci PM **Long-term follow-up of total hip replacement in patients with osteonecrosis** Orthop Clin North Am 1985; 16:757–769

Ficat noted that there are many factors which cause osteonecrosis. Whatever the pathological process, blockage of the osseous microcirculation with intramedullary stasis appears to be the common denominator. It is essential to diagnose osteonecrosis early by a bone scan while the hip is radiographically and clinically normal. Core decompression gives better results in Stage I than in Stage II. **Meyers** updated knowledge on the results of a pedicle graft of the quadratus femoris muscle for treatment of osteonecrosis of the femoral head. Results are good for early necrosis, Stages I and II, but poor for advanced necrosis, Stages III and IV. **Cornell** reviewed results of total hip arthroplasty in 33 consecutive patients with osteonecrosis from various causes. The revision rate at an average of 7 years of follow-up was 37% and the failure rate three times higher than that for degenerative joint disease. The higher failure rate is related to the underlying metabolic bone disease.

Caisson's Disease

McCallum RI, Waldor DN, Barnes R, Catto ME, Davidson JK, Fryer DI, Golding FC, Paton WDM **Bone lesions in compressed-air workers. Report of Decompression Sickness Panel, Medical Research Council** J Bone Joint Surg [Br] 1966;48B:207–235

Gregg PJ, Waldor DN **Scintigraphy versus radiology in the early diagnosis of experimental bone necrosis with special reference to Caisson disease of bone** J Bone Joint Surg [Br] 1980;62B:214–221

McCallum, in a classic article, described a radiographic investigation of 241 men who had worked in compressed air at pressures of up to 35 lb/in^2. Nineteen per cent had one or more lesions of aseptic necrosis of bone. In 10% the lesions were juxta-articular and therefore potentially disabling. Bone lesions were found to be directly related to the number of times a man had been decompressed, to the height of pressure at which he had worked and to attacks of bends for which treatment was given. **Gregg** noted that the early diagnosis of Caisson's disease of bone is hindered by the long delay which must elapse before an abnormality becomes apparent on a radiograph. Scintigraphy may have clinical value in Caisson's disease when a patient has pain but no clear evidence in radiographs of necrosis of bone.

Sickle-cell Disease

Golding JSR, MacIver JE, Went LN **The bone changes in sickle-cell anaemia and its genetic variants** J Bone Joint Surg [Br] 1959;41B:711–718

Iwegbu CG, Fleming AF **Avascular necrosis of the femoral head in sickle-cell disease: a series from the Guinea Savannah of Nigeria** J Bone Joint Surg [Br] 1985;67B:29–32

Hanker GJ, Amstutz HC **Osteonecrosis of the hip in the sickle-cell diseases: treatment and complications** J Bone Joint Surg [Am] 1988;70A:499–506

Mallouh A, Talab Y **Bone and joint infection in patients with sickle-cell disease** J Paediatr Orthop 1985;5:158–162

Golding surveyed knowledge on sickle-cell anaemia and its variants. The bone changes were divided into four groups, those due to hyperplasia, avascular necrosis, impaired growth and infection. The features of a crisis were described. Secondary osteomyelitis was common in sickle-cell anaemia and was often due to organisms of the salmonella group. **Iwegbu** discussed the incidence, clinical and radiographic characteristics of avascular necrosis of the femoral head in 899 patients with sickle-cell disease in Nigeria. The femoral head was involved in 29 patients; most were aged between 6 and 15 years at the onset of hip symptoms. The radiographic appearances varied widely, some being classified as a Perthes'-like lesion. **Hanker** described the results of hip arthroplasty in sickle-cell disease. They were not very satisfactory, with a high incidence of medical and surgical complications, particularly infection and mechanical and septic loosening. **Mallouh** described experience with 12 cases of bone and/or joint infection in patients with sickle-cell disease. Most were due to a salmonella organism. Differentiation from acute bone infarcts is difficult; an early diagnosis is necessary, using several blood cultures and needle aspiration.

Bone Dysplasias

The aim of this section is to provide references on the well-known dysplasias. We have avoided the rare syndromes and diseases.

Osteogenesis Imperfecta

Review Article

Cole WG **Osteogenesis imperfecta** In: Martin TJ, ed. Baillière's clinical endocrinology and metabolism: metabolic bone disease. London: Baillière Tindall, 1988;2:No.1:243–265

Cole provided a comprehensive recent chapter on all aspects of this condition. Four types are described: I blue sclera and autosomal dominant inheritance – the most common; II lethal perinatal – the most severe: III progressive and deforming, and IV white sclera with autosomal dominant inheritance. The collagen defects which lead to fragility are described with special reference to recent advances. The methods of diagnosis and their application at different ages are outlined, including diagnosis in utero. Treatment at all ages is debated, with special reference to fractures and deformities.

Treatment

Williams PF **Fragmentation and rodding in osteogenesis imperfecta** J Bone Joint Surg [Br] 1965;47B:23–31

Stockley I, Bell MJ, Sharrard WJW **The role of expanding intramedullary rods in osteogenesis imperfecta** J Bone Joint Surg [Br] 1989;71B:422–427

Morel G, Houghton GR **Pneumatic trouser splints in the treatment of severe osteogenesis imperfecta** Acta Orthop Scand 1982;52:547–552

Williams reported experience with 50 operations of fragmentation and rodding in the long bones with osteogenesis imperfecta. A modification of the original technique described by Sofield (1952) had been developed. The operation offered the patient a new life, virtually free of fractures. **Stockley** described the use of expanding intramedullary rods in 24 children. All revision operations were successful. Elongating intramedullary rods improve walking capacity, reduce the number of fractures and prevent deformity. **Morel** discussed the use of pneumatic orthoses in 12 patients. A closed osteotomy was followed by support in pneumatic trouser splints. The results of this conservative method compared favourably with those of multiple osteotomies and intramedullary rodding.

Book References

Smith R, Francis MJO, Houghton GR **The brittle bone syndrome – osteogenesis imperfecta.** London, Boston: Butterworths, 1983

Wynne Davies R, Hall CM, Apley AG **Osteogenesis imperfecta** In: Atlas of skeletal dysplasias. Edinburgh: Churchill Livingstone, 1985:411–430

Smith and his colleagues produced a comprehensive source for detailed reference on this subject. **Wynne Davies** has illustrated the clinical and radiological features.

Achondroplasia

Wynne Davies R, Walsh WK, Gormley J **Achondroplasia and hypochondroplasia: clinical variation and spinal stenosis** J Bone Joint Surg [Br] 1981; 63B:508–515

Aldegheri R, Trivella G, Renzi-Brivico L, Tessari G, Agostini S, Lavini F **Lengthening of the lower limbs in achondroplastic patients: a comparative study of four techniques** J Bone Joint Surg [Br] 1988;70B:69–73

Wynne Davies R, Hall CM, Apley AG **Achondroplasia** In: Atlas of skeletal dysplasias. Edinburgh: Churchill Livingstone, 1985:181–199

Wynne Davies provided a comprehensive study of the clinical and radiographic features of achondroplasia, based on a survey of 48 patients. The frequency of spinal stenosis and neurological complications was established in an unselected group of 27 achondroplastic and 12 hypochondroplastic patients aged 10 years and over. Only 3 of the former were free of symptoms but only 3 developed serious complications (11%). **Aldegheri** reported remarkable experience of lengthening by over 30% in 117 lower limbs in achondroplastic patients. Chondrodiatasis of the femur and callotasis of the tibia were the techniques which gave fewest complications. **Wynne Davies** illustrated the clinical and radiological features of this condition.

Dyschondroplasia (Ollier's Disease)

Shapiro F **Ollier's disease: an assessment of angular deformity, shortening and pathological fracture in 21 patients** J Bone Joint Surg [Am] 1982;64A: 95–103

Shapiro performed a retrospective review of 21 patients with Ollier's disease; this review is therefore a useful reference for this rare dysplasia. Typically, the disorder is unilateral. The femur and tibia are involved most frequently. Angular deformities are common, sometimes requiring osteotomy. Shortening is always present and may require epiphyseal arrest.

Hereditary Multiple Exostosis (Diaphyseal Aclasis)

Solomon L **Hereditary multiple exostosis** J Bone Joint Surg [Br] 1963;45B: 292–304

Shapiro F, Simon S, Glimcher MJ **Hereditary multiple exostoses: anthropometric, roentgenographic and clinical aspects** J Bone Joint Surg [Am] 1979;61A:815–824

Solomon, in a classic article, studied hereditary multiple exostosis in 56 patients and their relatives. The disease was inherited in approximately two-thirds of the cases. The possibility of malignant change in cartilage-capped exostosis was debated. More recently, **Shapiro** studied 32 patients and documented abnormalities in the forearm and proximal femur. Limb length discrepancies were common.

Fibrous Dysplasia

The Classic

Harris WH, Dudley HR, Barry RJ **The natural history of fibrous dysplasia: an orthopaedic pathological and roentgenographic study** J Bone Joint Surg [Am] 1962;44A:207–233

Harris studied the evolution of the skeletal lesions in a long-term follow-up of 37 cases of polyostotic fibrous dysplasia and 13 cases of monostotic fibrous dysplasia.

Enlargement of pre-existing lesions after puberty was not uncommon. The majority of pathological fractures heal with conservative therapy.

Clinical Studies

Stephenson RB, London MD, Hankin FM, Kaufer H **Fibrous dysplasia: an analysis of options for treatment** J Bone Joint Surg [Am] 1987;69A:400–409

Enneking WF, Gearen PF **Fibrous dysplasia of the femoral neck: treatment by cortical bone grafting** J Bone Joint Surg [Am] 1986;68A:1415–1422

Stephenson reviewed the results of treatment in 65 symptomatic lesions. Significant long-term morbidity is associated with this disease. Closed treatment of symptomatic lesions in the upper extremity provided a satisfactory functional outcome. In patients who are less than 18 years old, neither closed treatment nor curettage and bone grafting is adequate treatment for a symptomatic lesion in the lower extremity. Internal fixation should be strongly considered in these young patients. **Enneking** described and illustrated difficulties in the treatment of fibrous dysplasia of the femoral neck. The principle of cortical bone grafting without curettage, excision or internal fixation appears to be biologically and biomechanically sound.

Book Reference

Wynne Davies R, Hall CM, Apley AG **Polyostotic fibrous dysplasia** In: Atlas of skeletal dysplasias. Edinburgh: Churchill Livingstone, 1985:557–565

Wynne Davies illustrated the clinical and radiological features of this condition.

Neurofibromatosis

Review Article

Brill CB **Neurofibromatosis: clinical overview** Clin Orthop 1989;245:10–15

Brill summarised the protean clinical manifestations of neurofibromatosis. The disease is a relatively common genetic disorder; virtually all organ systems can be involved, either directly or through neural or vascular influences. Children and adults may be affected. The condition is inherited in autosomal dominant fashion. Benign or malignant tumours may develop.

The Spine

Hsu LCS, Lee PC, Leong JCY **Dystrophic spinal deformities in neurofibromatosis: treatment by anterior and posterior fusion** J Bone Joint Surg [Br] 1984;66B:495–499

Calvert PT, Edgar MA, Webb PJ **Scoliosis in neurofibromatosis: the natural history with and without operation** J Bone Joint Surg [Br] 1989;71B:246–251

Crawford AH **Pitfalls of spinal deformities associated with neurofibromatosis in children** Clin Orthop 1989;245:29–42

Hsu described the results of both anterior and posterior fusion for dystrophic spinal deformity in 13 patients. The morbidity rate was high in patients with angular kyphoscoliosis. Even anterior and posterior spinal fusion may fail to control the progressive deformity. **Calvert** reviewed 47 patients with neurofibromatosis and dystrophic spinal deformities. In many the natural history was observed. The most common pattern of deformity was a short angular thoracic scoliosis. Progression was usual, but the rate was variable and generally unpredictable. Severe dystrophic changes have a poor prognosis for deterioration. **Crawford** amplified the many problems which may be encountered in the treatment of spinal deformities associated with neurofibromatosis. Specialised CT myelography should be performed on all patients prior to surgical treatment. MRI assessment was recommended for any areas demonstrated to be suspect of previously unrecognised lesions. The most dangerous situation for the neurologically intact patient and the surgeon is the instrumentation and distraction of the spine in neurofibromatosis in the presence of unrecognised intraspinal lesions.

The Tibia

Boyd HB **The pathology and natural history of congenital pseudarthrosis of the tibia** Clin Orthop 1982;166:5–13

Murray HH, Lavell WW **Congenital pseudarthrosis of the tibia: a long-term follow-up study** Clin Orthop 1982;166:14–20

Boyd described a number of types of congenital pseudarthrosis of the tibia. Type II was the most common and had the worst prognosis. It was stated to be often associated with neurofibromatosis. The children were born with anterior bowing and hourglass constriction of the tibia. Spontaneous fracture or fracture following minor trauma commonly occurs before the age of 2 years. The bone ends are tapered, rounded and sclerotic, obliterating the medullary canal. **Murray** considered that stigmata of neurofibromatosis were present in about half the cases of his study of congenital pseudarthrosis of the tibia.

Book Reference

Wynne Davies R, Hall CM, Apley AG **Neurofibromatosis (von Recklinghausen's disease)** In: Atlas of skeletal dysplasias. Edinburgh: Churchill Livingstone, 1985:566–575

Wynne Davies described and illustrated the particular features of this condition.

The Upper Limb

Nerve Entrapment Syndromes

Review Articles

Chalmers J **Nerve compression syndromes** In: Lamb DW, Hooper G, Kuczynski K, eds. The practice of hand surgery. 2nd edn. Oxford: Blackwell Scientific Publications, 1989: 427-447

Howard FM **Controversies in nerve entrapment syndromes in the forearm and wrist** Orthop Clin North Am 1986;17:3:375-381

Chalmers produced a comprehensive recent review on nerve compression syndromes in the upper limb, including anatomy, clinical features, diagnostic tests and treatment. The large number of systemic and local conditions contributory to a carpal tunnel syndrome were tabled, with references to each. The clinical presentation and treatment of the pronator teres and anterior interosseous nerve syndromes were discussed. The causes of ulnar nerve compression both at the elbow and in relation to Guyon's canal were tabled. The arguments were marshalled for simple decompression as against anterior transposition for release of the ulnar nerve compression at the elbow. Subcutaneous and intramuscular beds are considered unsatisfactory and transposition deep to the flexor muscles is recommended. **Howard** considered controversies in relation to the five tunnels in the forearm and wrist where nerve entrapment may occur. A positive EMG report reinforces a clinical impression but if negative, does not exclude an entrapment syndrome.

Carpal Tunnel Syndrome

Green DP **Diagnostic and therapeutic value of carpal tunnel injection** J Hand Surg [Am] 1984;9-A:6:850-854

Payan J **Editorial: the carpal tunnel syndrome: can we do better?** J Hand Surg [Br] 1988;13-B:4:365-367

Seror P **Phalen's test in the diagnosis of carpal tunnel syndrome** J Hand Surg [Br] 1988;13-B:4:383–385

Altissimi M, Mancini GB **Surgical release of the median nerve under local anaesthesia for carpal tunnel syndrome** J Hand Surg [Br] 1988;13B:4:395–396

Hurst LC, Weissberg D, Carroll RE **The relationship of the double crush to carpal tunnel syndrome (an analysis of 1000 cases of carpal tunnel syndrome)** J Hand Surg [Br] 1985;10-B:2:202-204

Bradish CF **Carpal tunnel syndrome in patients on haemodialysis** J Bone Joint Surg [Br] 1985;67B:130-131

Pfeffer GB, Gelberman RH, Boyes JH, Rydevik B **The history of carpal tunnel syndrome** J Hand Surg [Br] 1988;13-B:28-34

Green described the results of 281 injections for carpal tunnel syndrome performed by one surgeon using the same technique. Injection is an effective, although usually transient, form of treatment. Eighty-one per cent of patients obtained good or complete relief, but in about one-half, (46%), sufficient symptoms recurred to warrant surgical treatment. A good response to injection is an excellent diagnostic and prognostic sign. **Payan**, in an editorial, discussed the various causes of dissatisfaction with the treatment of carpal tunnel syndrome and the value of electrodiagnosis. It may detect a co-existing unsuspected polyneuropathy, or assist where clinical diagnosis is in doubt. **Seror** analysed the value of the wrist flexion test of Phalen in 127 patients; the test was considered to be of real diagnostic and prognostic value but it was negative in 1 in 3 (34%) and positive in 20% of controls. **Altissimi** described experience of carpal tunnel release performed under local anaesthesia with a tourniquet in 124 patients. Only 1 patient had difficulty in tolerating the tourniquet, but in 18 cases the median nerve showed evidence of some damage caused by the needle or by injection of anaesthetic. At follow-up, no symptoms or signs related to this damage were found. **Hurst** studied a series of 1000 cases and showed a statistically significant incidence of bilaterality in patients with cervical arthritis. The double crush syndrome was debated; described by Upton in 1973, it stated that serial impingements upon a peripheral nerve can act in a cumulative manner to cause distal entrapment neuropathy. It is considered that the double crush syndrome predisposes to bilateral carpal tunnel syndrome and may be an important prognostic factor. **Bradish** reported eight cases of carpal tunnel syndrome, all of which developed in patients on haemodialysis for chronic renal failure. In each case, the arm involved had been used for a fistula. The cause of the syndrome is multifactorial but related to the sites of the arteriovenous fistulae. Decompression was effective and lasting. The paper by **Pfeffer** and his colleagues has been included for its special historical interest. He explained that, despite the common diagnosis of this condition now, as late as 1950 only 12 patients with operative release of the carpal ligament for idiopathic carpal tunnel syndrome had been reported. The confusion caused by the diverse manifestations of median nerve compression before the 1950s is discussed.

Pronator Teres Syndrome

Hartz CR, Linscheid RL, Gramse RR, Daube JR **The pronator teres syndrome: compressive neuropathy of the median nerve** J Bone Joint Surg [Am] 1981; 63A: 885–890

Hartz described a study of 39 patients with a clinical diagnosis of pronator teres syndrome seen during a 7-year period at the Mayo Clinic. The distinctive physical sign was tenderness over the proximal part of the pronator teres. EMG studies showed abnormality in only a few patients and localisation was rarely possible. Of 36 operations, 28 gave good or excellent results. The cause of failure was either inadequate decompression or missed diagnosis.

Anterior Interosseous Nerve Syndrome

Hill NA, Howard FM, Huffer BR **The incomplete anterior interosseous nerve syndrome** J Hand Surg [Am] 1985;10-A:4–16

Hill discussed 33 cases of an incomplete anterior interosseous nerve syndrome in which only the flexor pollicis longus or flexor digitorum profundus to the index finger was paralysed. The differential diagnosis is debated. The nerve is usually compressed by fibrous bands. Most patients will improve spontaneously; surgery is recommended, with exploration and neurolysis of the nerve for patients who show no improvement clinically or with repeat electromyography after 12 weeks of observation.

Ulnar Nerve Compression Syndrome

MacNicol MF **The results of operation for ulnar neuritis** J Bone Joint Surg [Br] 1979;61B:159–164

Gabel GT, Amadio PC **Reoperation for failed decompression of the ulnar nerve in the region of the elbow** J Bone Joint Surg [Am] 1990;72A:213–219

Shea JD, McClain EJ **Ulnar nerve compression syndromes at and below the wrist** J Bone Joint Surg [Am] 1969;51A:1095–1103

MacNicol compared the results of anterior transposition and simple release of the aponeurosis in patients with ulnar neuritis. The common abnormality was constriction by the flexor carpi ulnaris aponeurosis but in many, no abnormal pathology was found. Recovery was greatest when operation was performed within 3 months of onset of symptoms. It was recommended that release be restricted to patients with a short history and definite constriction. Anterior transposition is the operation of choice where no abnormality is seen, or where the nerve is compressed or dislocated proximal to the aponeurosis. **Gabel** reported his experience on 30 patients in a period of 6 years at the Mayo Clinic who had required revision for failed decompression of the ulnar nerve at the elbow. Most were revised by sub-muscular transposition of the nerve. At reoperation, all potential levels of compression must be released. The arcade of Struthers and also the medial intermuscular septum were frequently involved and it was stressed that the nerve is often compressed at several levels. The article represents a timely warning of poor results from ulnar nerve decompression at the elbow. Before operation, electrodiagnostic studies demonstrated at least one abnormality in 21 of the 30 patients. **Shea** provided a useful reference for ulnar nerve compression at the wrist. Three syndromes are presented and classified according to the local causes of compression. The sites are illustrated. Surgical decompression is recommended.

The Shoulder

Anterior Shoulder Pain

Review Article

Bayley I **Anterior shoulder pain** In: Catterall A, ed. Recent advances in ortho-paedics, 5. Edinburgh: Churchill Livingstone, 1987:123–152

Bayley provided a review of the many intrinsic causes of shoulder pain and their investigation. Symptoms of shoulder disease may be divided into four categories; pain, interference with mobility, weakness and mechanical derangement. There are short sections on rotator cuff impingement and painful arc syndromes, ruptures of the rotator cuff, acute and chronic and calcific tendonitis. Current knowledge of bicipital tendon pain is debated. The acromioclavicular joint is considered to be an underestimated source of anterior shoulder pain. Adhesive capsulitis or frozen shoulder is stated to be much overdiagnosed. Except for rheumatoid arthritis, glenohumeral joint arthritis is an uncommon cause of anterior shoulder pain.

Shoulder Arthroscopy

Ogilvie-Harris DJ, Wiley AM **Arthroscopic surgery of the shoulder: a general appraisal** J Bone Joint Surg [Br] 1986;68B:201–207

Rockwood CA **Editorial: shoulder arthroscopy** J Bone Joint Surg [Am] 1988; 70A:639–640

Gartsman GM **Mini-symposium: the shoulder (i) Shoulder arthroscopy** Curr Orthop 1990;4:4:218–224

Ogilvie-Harris summarised experience on 439 patients over a 10-year period. The study was retrospective and some of the conditions are difficult to define; presentation of results was therefore not precise. Arthroscopic surgery is safe and effective. It was useful in treating frozen shoulder, early osteoarthritis and isolated tears of the glenoid labrum. It was less useful in treating partial tears of the rotator cuff and tendonitis and was of no value in the treatment of complete tears of the cuff. Complications were rare. **Rockwood** discussed the use of arthroscopy both in the diagnosis and treatment of conditions of the shoulder. The use of the arthroscope for operative procedures is still in the developmental stage; whilst feasible, operative arthroscopy remains controversial. **Gartsman** provided an update on the technique and value of arthroscopy. It is useful in the diagnosis of difficult instability problems and in the recognition of unusual forms of shoulder arthritis. It is effective in the treatment of isolated stage II impingement and partial tears of the rotator cuff. Its value in adhesive capsulitis is limited, since there is soft-tissue contracture of the capsule; it has no value in the management of osteoarthritis.

Radiology

Magnetic Resonance Imaging

Iannotti JP, Zlatkin MB, Esterhai JL, Kressel HY, Dalinka MK, Spindler KP **Magnetic resonance imaging of the shoulder: sensitivity, specificity and predictive value** J Bone Joint Surg [Am] 1991;73A:17–29

Meyer AJF, Dalinki MK **Magnetic resonance imaging of the shoulder** Orthop Clin North Am 1990;21:3:497–513

Iannotti discussed the value of MRI of the shoulder in 91 patients. One hundred per cent sensitivity and 95% specificity was demonstrated in the diagnosis of complete tears of the rotator cuff. MRI is an excellent non-invasive tool in the diagnosis of lesions of the rotator cuff and glenohumeral instability. **Meyer** stressed that MRI was the only modality in which inflammatory changes in the tendons can be demonstrated.

Rotator Cuff Disorders

The Classic

Neer CS (II) **Anterior acromioplasty for the chronic impingement syndrome in the shoulder: a preliminary report** J Bone Joint Surg [Am] 1972;54A: 41–50

In 1972 **Neer** described the indications and technique of anterior acromioplasty. The treatment of impingement is to remove the anterior edge and under-surface of part of the acromion with the attached coracoacromial ligament.

Pathology – Clinical Features

Kessel L Watson M **The painful arc syndrome: clinical classification as a guide to management** J Bone Joint Surg [Br] 1977;59B:166–172

Fukuda H **Mini-symposium: the shoulder (ii) Shoulder impingement and rotator cuff disease** Curr Orthop 1990;4:4:225–232

Neer CS (II) **Impingement lesions** Clin Orthop 1983; 173:70–77

Kessel studied 97 patients suffering from painful arc syndrome. Those with lesions in the posterior part of the cuff, or anteriorly in the subscapularis tendon, resolved with injection of local anaesthetic and steroid. In the remainder, with lesions of the supraspinatus tendon, excision of the outer end of the clavicle and division of the coracoacromial ligament usually abolished the pain. **Fukuda** described three types of incomplete tear of the rotator cuff. The symptoms and signs of rotator cuff tears may be categorised into two groups, those caused by the inflammation and those caused by the torn tendon. **Neer** (II) (1983) described three stages of an impingement lesion: I oedema and haemorrhage; II fibrosis and tendonitis and III bone spurs and tendon rupture. An injection test was described to identify the lesion. Indications for arthrography were presented. Advantages of anterior acromioplasty over lateral acromionectomy include less deltoid detachment, better exposure and decompression of the supraspinatus.

Treatment

Cofield RH **Current concepts review: rotator cuff disease of the shoulder** J Bone Joint Surg [Am] 1985;67A:974–979

Neer CS (II), Marberry TA **On the disadvantages of radical acromionectomy** J Bone Joint Surg [Am] 1981;63A:416–419

Watson M **Major ruptures of the rotator cuff: the results of surgical repair in 89 patients** J Bone Joint Surg [Br] 1985;67B:618–624

Watson M **Rotator cuff function in the impingement syndrome** J Bone Joint Surg [Br] 1989;71B:361–366

Gartsman GM **Arthroscopic acromioplasty for lesions of the rotator cuff** J Bone Joint Surg [Am] 1990;72A:169–180

Cofield summarised knowledge of rotator cuff disease in 1985. Non-operative therapy may be effective but is not as consistently successful as was formerly believed. Anterior acromioplasty with limited detachment of the deltoid appears to be the most direct, least harmful and most effective procedure for rotator cuff tendonitis. The variable size and shape of tendon tears are discussed. The most direct and simple repair technique seems to be the best. **Neer** (1981) stressed the poor results of radical acromionectomy with persistent pain and weakened action of the deltoid. **Watson** (1985) discussed the results of repair of major ruptures of the rotator cuff. Poor results were associated with large cuff defects, preoperative steroid injections and deltoid weakness. The quality of the result improved for 2 years after surgery, but in those over 60 years old there was deterioration with time. Based on a study of 33 patients, **Watson** (1989) considered that excision arthroplasty of the acromioclavicular joint and anterior acromioplasty were highly effective for impingement under the acromium but only moderately effective when the impingement is under the acromioclavicular joint. **Gartsman** performed arthroscopic acromioplasty for a lesion of the rotator cuff in 165 patients; the operation consisted of acromioplasty, resection of the coracoacromial ligament and subacromial bursa and removal of osteophytes. The procedure was effective in the treatment of stage II impingement and partial tears. With complete tears results were inferior to those of traditional open repair, and arthroscopic decompression is not indicated.

Cuff-Tear Arthropathy

Neer CS (II), Craig EV, Fukuda H **Cuff-tear arthropathy** J Bone Joint Surg [Am] 1983;65A:1232–1244

Neer has drawn attention to the characteristics of a "new" condition in 26 patients. Following a massive tear of the rotator cuff, there is inactivity and disuse of the shoulder and instability, with the humeral head displaced upward causing subacromial impingement. The soft atrophic head may collapse and the condition is difficult to treat.

Instability

See **Dislocation of the shoulder joint** In: Ratliff AHC, Dixon JH, Magnussen PA, Young SK Selected references in orthopaedic trauma. London: Springer-Verlag, 1988:31–33

Hawkins RJ, Saddemi SR **Mini-symposium: the shoulder (iv) Shoulder instability** Current Orthop 1990;4:4:242–252

Mok DWH, Fogg AJB, Hokan R, Bayley JIL **The diagnostic value of arthroscopy in glenohumeral instability** J Bone Joint Surg [Br] 1990;72B: 698–700

Hawkins presented a classification of shoulder instability. Atraumatic dislocations occur in two situations: those with hyperlaxity and those who overuse their shoulders. The patient with a recurrent subluxation who has never had a documented dislocation can present a diagnostic challenge. Methods of assessment of stability are discussed, including apprehension testing. The relative merits of the Putti–Platt, Magnuson–Stack, Bristow and Bankart procedures are debated. Atraumatic instability differs from traumatic instability since there is usually no Bankart lesion. Problems of posterior instability are debated. **Mok** described the results of 166 shoulder arthroscopies performed in patients with symptoms of subluxation but no firm evidence of dislocation and no definite diagnosis. Arthroscopy was useful in establishing the pathogenesis and direction of instability.

Arthroplasty

Clinical Studies

Neer CS (II), Watson KC, Stanton FJ **Recent experience in total shoulder replacement** J Bone Joint Surg [Am] 1982;64A:319–337

Lettin AWF, Copeland SA, Scales JT **The Stanmore total shoulder replacement** J Bone Joint Surg [Br] 1982;64B:47–51

Cofield RH **Total shoulder arthroplasty with the Neer prosthesis** J Bone Joint Surg [Am] 1984;66A:899–906

Barrett WP, Franklin JL, Jackins SE, Wyss CR, Matsen FA (III) **Total shoulder arthroplasty** J Bone Joint Surg [Am] 1987;69A:865–872

Kelly IG, Foster RS, Fisher WD **Neer total shoulder replacement in rheumatoid arthritis** J Bone Joint Surg [Br] 1987;69B:723–726

Browne AO, McCann PD **The current status of shoulder arthroplasty** Curr Orthop 1988;2:2:94–98

Neer presented experience using an unconstrained implant based on a study of 194 operations observed for a minimum of 2 years. Neither loss of bone nor a deficient rotator cuff was regarded as a contraindication to replacement. Function depends on meticulous reconstruction. Only 4 patients had not benefited and loosening did not occur. The results of 50 replacements using the Stanmore prosthesis are described by **Lettin**. Nine patients were eventually left with an excisional arthroplasty. The Stanmore prosthesis will relieve pain and restore a functional range of movement in the majority of severely disabled patients, but improvement was inconsistent and sometimes disappointing. **Cofield**'s paper provides another surgeon's experience of the use of the Neer prosthesis; similar excellent results were achieved although there was a greater incidence of loosening. The glenoid component may require improvement. **Barrett**, in a prospective study of 50 replacements stressed the significant relief of pain which could be obtained but emphasised the need for training for performance of these operations. **Kelly** discussed the special problems of shoulder replacement in rheumatoid arthritis based on 42 cases observed for up to 5 years. Involvement of the rotator cuff is common and explains the failure to regain more than a moderate range of elevation. Nevertheless, gratifying results have been obtained with good relief of pain and improved function. Non-constrained shoulder arthroplasty does merit a place in the surgical management of rheumatoid arthritis. **Browne** noted the low incidence of loosening with cemented non-constrained shoulder replacement. The importance of both surgical technique and postoperative rehabilitation was stressed. In rheumatoid arthritis, severe destruction of the rotator cuff compromises the functional result. With disease of both shoulder and elbow, shoulder arthroplasty should be considered before elbow arthroplasty; many patients benefit sufficiently from shoulder arthroplasty to defer elbow surgery. A constrained joint like the Stanmore is no longer recommended because of the high rate of loosening. Results are poor from interpositional arthroplasty with silastic implant.

Rheumatoid Arthritis

Clinical Studies

Crossan JF, Vallance R **The shoulder joint in rheumatoid arthritis** In: Bayley I, Kessel L, eds. Shoulder surgery. Berlin: Springer-Verlag, 1982:131–139

Kelly IG **Surgery of the rheumatoid shoulder** Ann Rheum Dis 1990; 49:Suppl 2:824–829

Kelly IG, Foster RS, Fisher WD **Neer total shoulder replacement in rheumatoid arthritis** J Bone Joint Surg [Br] 1987;69B:723–726

Review Article

Beddow FH **Surgical management of the rheumatoid shoulder** In: Beddow FH, ed. Surgical management of rheumatoid arthritis. London: Wright, 1988:55–67

Crossan described progressive radiological grades of involvement of the joint with chronic proximal subluxation of the humeral head in severe cases. A dramatic deterioration in function occurs in end-stage disease,with appreciable pain. **Kelly** (1990) discussed patterns of joint disease, sites of pain and involvement of the acromioclavicular joint. The value of various surgical procedures to the acromioclavicular joint, the subacromial region and the shoulder joint are debated. Synovectomy and arthrodesis are rarely of value. **Kelly** (1987), discussed the special problems of shoulder replacement in rheumatoid arthritis based on experience of 42 cases observed for 5 years. Involvement of the rotator cuff is almost universal and explains the failure to regain more than a moderate range of elevation. Nevertheless, gratifying results have been obtained with good relief of pain and improved function. Non-constrained shoulder arthroplasty does merit a place in the surgical management of rheumatoid arthritis. **Beddow** considered that the use of arthrodesis in the treatment of rheumatoid shoulder has never been popular because of the polyarthritic nature of the disease, but it has a place when there is a painful fibrous ankylosis. The value of excision arthroplasty, interposition arthroplasty and prosthetic replacement are debated. It is stressed that shoulder replacement is a technically difficult operation since there is often poor bone stock on the glenoid side and defective musculature.

Frozen Shoulder

Clinical Studies

Haines JF, Hargadon EJ **Manipulation as the primary treatment of the frozen shoulder** J R Coll Surg Edinb 1982;271–275

Kessel L, Bayley I, Young A **The frozen shoulder** Br J Hosp Med 1981;25: 334–349

Haines discussed the value of manipulation based on a retrospective study of 78 cases. He considered manipulation to be safe, satisfactory and effective. **Kessel** considered that the diagnosis of frozen shoulder should be reserved for patients with spontaneous shoulder pain, restriction of glenohumeral movements, no general illness and normal radiographs. Arthrographic studies confirm that the joint capacity is considerably reduced; there is evidence of disease of the joint capsule with fibrosis. The evidence for an immunological basis for a frozen shoulder remains scanty. When combined with physiotherapy, manipulation may shorten the total duration of the disease; it should be performed when the acute phase has subsided. The authors have noted the small number of papers on this ill-defined condition.

Book Reference

Rowe CR, Leffert RD **Idiopathic chronic adhesive capsulitis ("frozen shoulder")** In: Rowe CR, ed. The shoulder. New York: Churchill Livingstone, 1988:155–163

Rowe considered that chronic adhesive capsulitis is one of the least understood of problems of the shoulder. It is usually a self-limited syndrome which passes through three distinct phases called respectively, the freezing, the frozen and the thawing. The possibilities of treatment are debated.

The Elbow Joint

Tennis Elbow

Nirschl RP, Pettrone FA **Tennis elbow: the surgical treatment of lateral epicondylitis** J Bone Joint Surg [Am] 1979;61A:832–839

Roles NC, Maudsley RH **Radial tunnel syndrome: resistant tennis elbow as a nerve entrapment** J Bone Joint Surg [Br] 1972;54B:499–508

Heyse-Moore GH **Resistant tennis elbow** J Hand Surg 1984;9B:1:64–66

Controversy has centred on the pathophysiology of this condition. Tennis elbow rarely requires surgical treatment. **Nirschl** described the pathology in 82 patients requiring operation. There was immature fibroblastic and vascular infiltration of the origin of extensor carpi radialis brevis. A specific technique was employed including excision of the lesion and repair. There was an overall improvement in a large percentage of patients. The treatment of tennis elbow by surgery remains controversial. **Roles** described treatment of resistant cases by decompression of the radial nerve in front of the elbow, believing an entrapment neuropathy to be present. An operation is described and illustrated to explore the nerve through an anterior approach in 36 patients. **Heyse-Moore** studied 50 cases of resistant tennis elbow; 37 were treated by lengthening the tendon of extensor carpi radialis brevis and 13 by decompression of the radial tunnel. The results of surgery were very similar in the two groups. Surgical division of the fibrous arch of the superficial part of supinator will relieve tension on the lateral epicondyle, thus allowing decompression of the radial nerve. There was no clinical or electrical evidence of radial nerve entrapment in resistant tennis elbow.

The Rheumatoid Elbow

Synovectomy

Porter BB, Richardson C, Vainio K **Rheumatoid arthritis of the elbow: the results of synovectomy** J Bone Joint Surg [Br] 1974;56B:427–437

Brumfield RH, Resnick CT **Synovectomy of the elbow in rheumatoid arthritis** J Bone Joint Surg [Am] 1985;67A:16–20

Tulp NJA, Winia WPCA **Synovectomy of the elbow in rheumatoid arthritis: long-term results** J Bone Joint Surg [Br] 1989;71B:664–666

Souter WA **Surgery for rheumatoid arthritis I. Upper limb: surgery of the elbow** Curr Orthop 1989;3:9–13

Porter reviewed the results of a radical synovectomy performed on 154 elbows in the Rheumatism Foundation Hospital in Finland. The detailed technique, with two incisions as advocated by Vainio, was described. The paper indicates the problems of assessment of results of synovectomy. Seventy per cent of the patients were pleased with the outcome. Good results were likely to be short-lived when the disease was far advanced by the time of operation. **Brumfield** described the results in 35 patients when synovectomy and resection of the radial head was performed for advanced disease (stage III or IV). He concluded that this operation was not contraindicated for relief of pain but no improvement in movement could be expected. Long-term results of synovectomy were described by **Tulp**. Follow-up was over 6 years. Results were satisfactory in 67%, with no deterioration. In this study there was no significant difference between the results of the early and late synovectomies. For this reason, synovectomy is recommended even in destroyed joints instead of prosthetic replacement. **Souter** noted that 50% of patients with long-standing rheumatoid disease will show evidence of elbow involvement. Five grades of radiological deterioration can be recognised. Routine radial head excision is not advised as an adjunct to synovectomy in early grades of this disease, i.e., grades I and II. Synovectomy should not be regarded as a definitive and lasting solution for the rheumatoid elbow, but rather as buying valuable time before more radical surgery may have to be undertaken. Synovectomy remains a powerful weapon for treatment of early rheumatoid disease.

Total Elbow Arthroplasty

Historical

Souter WA **Metallic hinge arthroplasty in the rheumatoid elbow** J Bone Joint Surg [Br] 1973;55B:874

Morrey BF, Bryan RS **Infection after total elbow arthroplasty** J Bone Joint Surg [Am] 1983;65A:330–338

In 1973 **Souter** reported on a series of 25 metallic hinge arthroplasties of the elbow performed in 20 patients with a relatively short follow-up. With time, deterioration in results had occurred. There was a high incidence of loosening of the humeral component, associated with thinning of the surrounding cortex. It was suggested that hinge arthroplasty should be used only in very disabled elderly patients who were unlikely to subject the implant to excessive use. There was a need for development of prostheses which allow for rotary stress. **Morrey** described deep sepsis in 9% of 156 elbow-replacement procedures. The high incidence of this complication should act as a warning to the hazardous nature of an elbow replacement procedure in rheumatoid arthritis. Compared with the hip and the knee, elbow arthroplasty still presents many difficult problems.

Review Article

Goldberg VM, Figgie AE (III), Inglis AE, Figgie MP **Current concepts review: total elbow arthroplasty** J Bone Joint Surg [Am] 1988;70A:778–783

Goldberg considered that elbow arthroplasty has now evolved from a single axis hinge joint to a complex unconstrained arthroplasty. The primary indication is relief of pain with a secondary indication being restoration of stability. Currently available implants are discussed, including resurfacing and semi-constrained. Technical considerations are debated. When techniques are satisfactory, 90% of patients have achieved a good or excellent result with resurfacing prostheses. Revision arthroplasty presents major problems, often with poor bone stock and fibrosis. Revision may be necessary for septic loosening, aseptic failure or dislocation.

Clinical Studies

Souter WA **Surgery for rheumatoid arthritis: I. Upper limb surgery of the elbow** Curr Orthop 1989;3:9–13

Roper BA, Tuke M, O'Riordan SM, Bulstrode CJ **A new unconstrained elbow: a prospective review of 60 replacements** J Bone Joint Surg [Br] 1986; 68B:566–569

Weiland AJ, Weiss APC, Wills RP, Russell Moore J **Capitellocondylar total elbow replacement: a long-term follow-up study** J Bone Joint Surg [Am] 1989; 71A:217–222

Figgie MP, Inglis AE, Mow CS, Figgie AE (III) **Total elbow arthroplasty for complete ankylosis of the elbow** J Bone Joint Surg [Am] 1989;71A:513–520

Souter described the emergence of a second generation of elbow implants. One of the main factors in producing loosening was the high torsional forces generated during ordinary activities of living. HDP bushing of any hinge implant is mandatory and hinges should only be semi-constrained or floppy. Elbow arthroplasty is now on the threshold of achieving a secure place in the rheumatoid surgeon's repertoire. One year after surgery, 92% of 112 cases where the Souter–Strathclyde prosthesis had been inserted had no pain. The complications of the operation are discussed. **Roper** reviewed results of 60 unconstrained elbow replacements of a new design followed prospectively for 3–9 years. Fifty per cent had excellent relief of pain and return of function but 27% had had major complications requiring removal and revision of the prosthesis. **Weiland** described the results of 40 total elbow replacements using a capitellocondylar prosthesis. The average length of follow-up was 7 years. Movements improved considerably except for extension. To date, none of these prostheses have shown any clinical evidence of loosening, but there was radiographic evidence of radiolucent lines in 10 elbows. **Figgie** described the results of 16 patients with ankylosed elbows and insertion of a total elbow arthroplasty. Semi-constrained prostheses are recommended in these cases since the supportive ligaments are not functional. Functional improvement is possible but considerable preoperative planning is required and the use of a custom-made semi-constrained prosthesis is often necessary.

Revision Elbow Arthroplasty

Morrey BF & Bryan RS **Revision total elbow arthroplasty** J Bone Joint Surg [Am] 1987;69A:523–532

Morrey recorded experience over a 10-year period with 33 revision total elbow arthroplasties. The majority were performed for rheumatoid arthritis but some followed post-traumatic arthritis. Data from this study indicated that reimplantation is a viable option for the revision of a failed total elbow arthroplasty, but it was suggested that young patients who have post-traumatic arthritis should not undergo a total joint replacement. There was sometimes appreciable loss of bone stock in the distal part of the humerus, depending on the nature of the lesion and the design of the initial prosthesis.

THE HAND

Congenital Abnormalities

Lamb DW **Congenital malformation of the upper limb** Curr Orthop 1990; 4:263–270

Lamb provided a useful general reference to congenital abnormalities of the upper limb. The management of the radial club hand is summarised. The deformity is ugly and progresses during growth. Splinting the wrist straight from an early age is advisable. If there is active elbow flexion to 90°, the wrist deformity should be corrected. The most satisfactory operation is centralisation of the carpus over the lower end of the ulna. It is unlikely that most surgeons will have much personal exposure to or experience in the management of these conditions and therefore the authors have not studied references in depth. Lamb stressed the need for special clinics and skills for the management of these complex problems.

Stenosing Tenosynovitis

Digital

Rhoades CE, Gelberman RH, Manjarris JF **Stenosing tenosynovitis of the fingers and thumb: results of a prospective trial of steroid injection and splinting** Clin Orthop 1984;190:236–238

Thorpe AP **Results of surgery for trigger finger** J Hand Surg [Br] 1988;13B: 199–201

Rhoades performed a prospective study of the value of steroid injection. In 72% of digits the outcome was successful, but some were only temporarily improved. The patient with less than 4 months of symptoms responded most favourably. **Thorpe** reviewed 43 patients and found that 60% of operations were "completely successful". However, 15 operations led to complications, including recurrence of clicking and nerve damage. Some were performed by junior surgeons.

De Quervain's Disease

Faithfull DK, Lamb DW **De Quervain's disease – a clinical review** The Hand 1971;3:23–30

Book Reference

Hooper G **Stenosing tenosynovitis and de Quervain's tenosynovitis** In: Lamb DW, Hooper G, Kuczynski K, eds. The practice of hand surgery. 2nd edn. Oxford: Blackwell Scientific Publications, 1989: 649–650

Faithfull carried out a retrospective clinical study of 80 patients. Results of treatment, both conservative and surgical, were evaluated. This is a disease predominantly of females between the ages of 40 and 70. Surgery is a quick, easy and reliable method of treatment. **Hooper** reviewed both conditions; care must be taken to avoid damage to the terminal sensory branches of the radial nerve.

Dupuytren's Disease

Aetiology

Ling RSM **The genetic factor in Dupuytren's disease** J Bone Joint Surg [Br] 1963;45B:709–718

Noble J, Heathcote JG, Cohen H **Diabetes mellitus in the aetiology of Dupuytren's disease** J Bone Joint Surg [Br] 1984;66B:322–325

Murrell GAC, Francis MJO, Howlett CR **Dupuytren's contracture: fine structure in relation to aetiology** J Bone Joint Surg [Br] 1989;71B:367–373

Ling studied the families of 50 patients with Dupuytren's disease. He found that familial occurrence was considerably higher than previously reported and that genetic factors are of importance in the pathogenesis. A single gene, behaving as a Mendelian dominant, is likely to be involved. **Noble** showed a 42% incidence of Dupuytren's disease in adult diabetics. The incidence was highest in older patients with a long history but was not related to the severity of the diabetes. The disease was mild with a benign prognosis, rarely needing surgery. **Murrell** compared the fine structure of palmar fascia from areas of Dupuytren's contracture with that from patients with carpal tunnel syndrome. The ultrastructure of fibroblasts appeared identical but there was a difference in fibroblast density; it was suggested that oxygen free-radicals cause necrosis and fibroblastic proliferation.

Pathogenesis

Brickley-Parsons D, Glimcher MJ, Smith RJ, Albin R, Adams JP **Biochemical changes in the collagen of the palmar fascia in patients with Dupuytren's disease** J Bone Joint Surg [Am] 1981;63A:787–797

Badalamente MA, Stern L, Hurst LC **The pathogenesis of Dupuytren's contracture: contractile mechanisms of the myofibroblasts** J Hand Surg [Am] 1983;8A:235–243

Brickley-Parsons studied palmar fascia from 400 patients and 100 controls biochemically. Modifications of the collagen in Dupuytren's disease did not appear to be the cause of the contracture but represented changes similar to rapidly synthesised new collagen seen in the active stages of wound repair. The biochemical abnormalities may account for the high rate of recurrence after surgical excision of the visibly affected area. **Badalamente** investigated fascia from 20 patients by light and electron microscopic histochemical techniques. Dupuytren's nodules were found to contain large numbers of modulated fibroblasts called myofibroblasts. Residual post-surgical contracture and recurrence appeared to be related to the number of nodular myofibroblasts present.

Long-term Results

Honner R, Lamb DW, James JIP **Dupuytren's contracture: long-term results after fasciectomy** J Bone Joint Surg [Br] 1971;53B:240–246

Honner studied the results in 138 hands operated on for Dupytren's contracture. Contracture of the metacarpophalangeal joint can be expected to respond well to operation, whereas the outlook for contracture of the proximal interphalangeal joint was generally poor. A gradual increase in this contracture occurred with time.

Surgical Treatment

Strickland JW, Bassett RL **The isolated digital cord in Dupuytren's contracture: anatomy and clinical significance** J Hand Surg [Am] 1985;10A: 118–124

Carr TL **Local radical fasciectomy for Dupuytren's contracture.** The Hand 1974;6:40–49

Tonkin MA, Burke FD, Varian JPW **Dupuytren's contracture: a comparative study of fasciectomy and dermofasciectomy in 100 patients** J Hand Surg 1984; 9B:156–162

Lubahn JD, Lister GD, Wolfe T **Fasciectomy and Dupuytren's disease: a comparison between the open palm technique and wound closure** J Hand Surg [Am] 1984;9A:53–58

Schneider LH, Hankin FM, Eisenberg T **Surgery of Dupuytren's disease: a review of the open palm method** J Hand Surg [Am] 1986;11A:23–27

Strickland outlined the pathological anatomy of isolated digital involvement in Dupuytren's disease, based on experience with 37 digits. The article is useful in preoperative planning. **Carr** described the results of local radical fasciectomy based on a study of 250 patients. There was a recurrence of disease within the field of operation in 25% and extension of the disease to other areas in 28%. **Tonkin** studied the results of 128 operations comparing those with primary skin closure and those with a full-thickness skin graft. The recurrence rate after surgery was 46%. Skin excision and replacement following fasciectomy prevented any appreciable recurrence of Dupuytren's tissue. Skin replacement did not jeopardise hand function. **Lubahn** analysed 153 patients treated surgically. Complications were fewer and motion better in the open palm group. The open palm technique may be most applicable for patients with extensive disease. By leaving the palmar wound open, skin closure under tension and risk of damage to the blood supply was avoided. **Schneider** noted the minimal postoperative morbidity with the open palm technique, but long-term follow-up revealed a significant rate of recurrence (32%) and extension (48%). The open palm method does not modify the long-term results.

Book Reference

Hueston JT, Tubiana R, eds. **Dupuytren's disease**, 2nd English edn. London: Churchill Livingstone, 1985

This monograph contains a number of authoritative chapters, including contributions concerning the anatomy (McGrouther, pages 38–54) and the open palm technique (McCash, pages 136–141). Skoog (pages 184–192) believed that the essential pathology involves the superficial longitudinal bands and not the underlying transverse palmar ligament. Operative difficulties are discussed by Michon (pages 177–183) and complications of fasciectomy by Tubiana (pages 197–199).

Kienbock's Disease

Clinical Studies

Alexander AH, Lichtman DM **Kienbock's disease** Orthop Clin North Am 1986;17:3:461–472

Almquist EE **Kienbock's disease** Clin Orthop 1986;202:68–78

Sundberg SB, Linscheid RL **Kienbock's disease: results of treatment with ulnar lengthening** Clin Orthop 1984;187:43–51

Kristensen SS, Soballe K **Kienbock's disease – the influence of arthrosis on ulnar variance measurements** J Hand Surg [Br] 1987;12-B:3:301–305

Palmer A **Editorial: Kienbock's disease - the influence of arthrosis on ulnar variance determination** J Hand Surg [Br] 1987;12-B:3:291–293

Nakamura R, Imaeda T, Miura T **Radial shortening for Kienbock's disease: factors affecting the operative result** J Hand Surg [Br] 1990;15-B:1:40–45

Alexander in 1986 provided a concise recent review of the controversies concerning Kienbock's disease. The four stages of progression are described and illustrated by Lichtman, and the significance of ulnar variance is debated. Treatment options are discussed in detail. Immobilisation is recommended for Stage I; for Stage II a revascularisation procedure or ulnar lengthening/radial shortening may be performed, especially if there is significant ulnar variance. A silicone arthroplasty is the treatment of choice for Stage III and for Stage IV a salvage procedure. The paper by **Almquist** describes various procedures, including radial shortening and ulnar lengthening and different types of localised intercarpal fusion. The Mayo Clinic experience of ulnar lengthening is described by **Sundberg**. The patients were well satisfied with relief of pain but the follow-up was short. This method of treatment is often recommended as the initial treatment since it does not violate the carpus or 'burn any bridges'. **Kristensen** measured the difference in ulnar variance between diseased and unaffected wrists in 38 patients with unilateral disease. He considered there was no difference in measurements in patients without arthrosis. With increasing arthrosis, there was an apparent pseudo-lengthening of the radius. He concluded that this was a consequence of the disease and that negative ulnar variance did not cause Kienbock's disease. **Palmer**, in an editoral, debated the evidence for this contention. **Nakamura** described the operative results of radial shortening in 23 patients and noted that age was a principal factor, unsatisfactory results being obtained in patients over 30 years of age. The risk of ulnar wrist pain was increased when the radius was shortened by more than 4 mm. Clearly, the treatment of Kienbock's disease remains controversial.

Osteoarthritis – First Carpometacarpal Joint

Gervis WH A review of excision of the trapezium for osteoarthritis of the trapeziometacarpal joint after 25 years J Bone Joint Surg [Br] 1973;55B: 56–57

Burton RI Basal joint implant arthroplasty in osteoarthritis: indications, techniques, pitfalls and problems Hand Clin 1987;3:473–485

Gervis recorded a practical appraisal of the value of excision of the trapezium. Results were considered to be entirely satisfactory. **Burton** concluded that implant arthroplasty is a valuable surgical procedure for some patients with basal joint arthritis of the thumb. It appears to be most useful in patients with a low-demand osteoarthritis, and in rheumatoid arthritis. The associated soft-tissue reconstruction is of paramount importance in determining success; instability may be a problem. The long-term results described by Swanson are discussed (J Hand Surg [Am] 1981;6:125–141).

The Rheumatoid Hand

The Classic

Swanson AB Flexible implant arthroplasty for arthritic finger joints: rationale, technique and results of treatment J Bone Joint Surg [Am] 1972; 54A:435–455

In 1972, **Swanson** described the development of silicone implants as an arthroplasty for metacarpophalangeal and interphalangeal joints, using the concept of fixation by encapsulation. The technique, results and complications were described, based on personal experience of the author and in patients treated by surgeons in many clinics who participated in a Field Clinic Study. Good results were achieved, with an impressive range of flexion and correction of deformity.

Review Articles

Nalebuff EA Surgery for rheumatoid arthritis: 1. Upper limb: surgery of the wrist and hand Curr Orthop 1989;3:14–20

Souter WA **Rheumatoid arthritis – general principles of surgical management.** In: Lamb DW, Hooper G, Kuczynski K, eds. The practice of hand surgery. 2nd edn. Oxford: Blackwell Scientific Publications, 1989:532–548

Mannerfelt L **Editorial: surgery of the rheumatoid hand: consensus and controversy** J Hand Surg [Br] 1989;14B:3:259–260

Nalebuff provided a concise review of the use of surgery, including joint synovectomy, tenosynovectomy, tendon surgery, arthroplasty and arthrodesis. Most surgeons believe that some benefit is derived from synovectomy, although controlled studies are impossible to perform and the subject is therefore controversial. Synovial proliferation may produce different clinical patterns on the flexor and extensor aspects of the hand, but responds well to surgical excision. The merits of arthroplasty and arthrodesis are debated. There continues to be an important place in surgery of the rheumatoid hand for joint fusion to correct deformity, relieve pain and provide stability. **Souter** summarised the guiding principles of surgical management, stressing the importance of tailoring the surgical programme to the needs of the individual patient. Deformity is an indication for surgery only if accompanied by pain or loss of function. The surgical programme should be staged, starting with simple successful operations. The treatment of extensor and flexor tenosynovitis and their complications are debated in detail. **Mannerfelt** discussed the value of early synovectomy and later bony surgery, especially arthrodesis of the wrist and of the metacarpophalangeal joint of the thumb.

The Wrist

Vicar AJ, Burton RI **Surgical management of the rheumatoid wrist – fusion or arthroplasty?** J Hand Surg [Am] 1986;11A:6:790–797

Kobus RJ, Turner RH **Wrist arthrodesis for treatment of rheumatoid arthritis** J Hand Surg [Am] 1990; 15A:4:541–546

Koka R, D'Arcy JC **Stabilisation of the wrist in rheumatoid disease** J Hand Surg [Br] 1989;14B:3:288–290

Swanson AB, Swanson G de G, Maupin BK **Flexible implant arthroplasty of the radiocarpal joint – surgical technique and long-term study** Clin Orthop 1984;187:94–106

Brase DW, Millender LH **Failure of silicone rubber wrist arthroplasty in rheumatoid arthritis** J Hand Surg [Am] 1986;11A:2:175–183

Vicar compared the results of arthrodesis and arthroplasty. Arthrodesis showed 97% excellent or good results with decreased pain, but some complained of loss of dexterity. In the arthroplasty group, 78% were good or excellent. The complication rate was higher (25%). **Kobus** described the results of arthrodesis with the Millender–Nalebuff technique (JBJS [Am] 1973; 1026) with 97% excellent or good. The operation is a dependable procedure with a high degree of success. The most common complication was pain from the tip of the Steinman pin. A neutral position of the wrist with slight ulnar deviation is functional. **Koka** recommended simple stabilisation of the wrist using internal fixation with an intramedullary Rush nail. The operation is simple and external immobilisation is unnecessary. **Swanson**, in 1984, described the technique of silicone arthroplasty, based on experience of 181 implant procedures. Stable pain-free motion was obtained in the majority of cases and complications were stated to be infrequent. However, **Brase** found 20% had fractured and an additional 5% required revision. He advised that consideration should be given to alternative methods of treatment.

Silicone Synovitis

Peimer CA, Medige J, Eckert BS, Wright JR, Howard CS **Reactive synovitis after silicone arthroplasty** J Hand Surg [Am] 1986;11A:5:624–638

Carter PR, Benton LJ, Dysert PA **Silicone rubber carpal implants: a study of the incidence of late osseous complications** J Hand Surg [Am] 1986;11A:5:639–644

The papers by **Peimer** and **Carter** reflect increased interest in the reactions to silicone. **Peimer** described the erosive osteolysis which occurred with progressive bone destruction. Silicone microparticles was the result of implant degeneration. The synovitis and destruction were arrested by the removal of the implant and synovectomy. **Carter** reviewed experience of 53 silicone implants. Wear was more common than suggested by isolated case reports. The use of carpal implants in healthy vigorous young patients is questionable. Both these authors stress the need for careful follow-up of these patients.

Surgery

1. Flexor Tendons

Stanley JK **Surgery of flexor tendons** In: FH Beddow, ed. Surgical management of rheumatoid arthritis. London: Wright, 1988:86–91

Mannerfelt L, Norman O **Attrition ruptures of flexor tendons in rheumatoid arthritis caused by bony spurs in the carpal tunnel: a clinical and radiological study** J Bone Joint Surg [Br] 1969;51B:270–277

Disease affecting the flexor tendons occurs in 60–70% of patients with rheumatoid arthritis. **Stanley** discussed treatment for involvement of the wrist, palm and digital flexor sheath, including synovitis, trigger thumb, trigger finger and tendon rupture. **Mannerfelt** described the presentation and cause of flexor tendon rupture in 25 cases. These were attributed equally to attrition and synovial invasion. Bony spurs can cause attrition rupture of flexor tendons, especially the flexor pollicis longus.

---

2. Extensor Tendons and Dorsum of Wrist

Stanley JK **Surgery of the wrist and extensor tendons** In: FH Beddow, ed. Surgical management of rheumatoid arthritis. London: Wright 1988:92–95

Abernethy PJ, Dennyson WG **Decompression of the extensor tendons at the wrist in rheumatoid arthritis** J Bone Joint Surg [Br] 1979;61B:64–68

Newman RJ **Excision of the distal ulna in patients with rheumatoid arthritis** J Bone Joint Surg [Br] 1987;69B:203–206

Magnussen PA, Harvey FJ, Tonkin MA **Extensor indicis proprius transfer for rupture of the extensor pollicis longus tendon** J Bone Joint Surg [Br] 1990;72B:881–883

Stanley reviewed experience in the exposure and treatment of extensor tendon pathology on the dorsum of the wrist. The management of extensor tendon rupture, sometimes multiple, is debated. **Abernethy** discussed the treatment of the common dorsal tenosynovitis of the wrist. Simple decompression of the extensor tendons had been carried out in 54 patients and the synovitis usually resolved. It was considered that the clinical result of decompression compared favourably with the widely accepted operation of dorsal synovectomy. **Newman** described the results of excision of the distal ulna in 34 wrists in patients with chronic rheumatoid arthritis. There was a marked relief of symptoms especially that of pain. Nevertheless, function of the upper limb was improved in only 25%. The results of extensor indicis transfer for extensor pollicis rupture are described by **Magnussen**. Although only some of the cases were for rheumatoid arthritis, the paper is included as a useful review of the subject. The operation is simple and reliable, with few complications. Satisfactory extension of the thumb is restored.

---

3. Metacarpophalangeal Joints of the Fingers

Swanson AB, Swanson G de G **Arthroplasty in the rheumatoid hand** In: Lamb DW, Hooper G, Kuczynski K, eds. The practice of hand surgery. 2nd edn. Oxford: Blackwell Scientific Publications, 1989:565–572

Bieber EJ, Weiland AJ, Volenec-Dowling S **Silicone-rubber implant arthroplasty of the metacarpophalangeal joints for rheumatoid arthritis** J Bone Joint Surg [Am] 1986;68A:206–209

Swanson updated previous publications and particularly stressed patient selection and indications for metacarpophalangeal arthroplasty. These include stiff joints, severe joint destruction or subluxation and ulnar drift not correctable by surgery of soft tissues alone. At surgery, tight ulnar intrinsics must be released, the volar subluxation corrected and the extensor tendons relocated. The postoperative splintage is stressed. **Bieber** discussed results of arthroplasty of 210 joints observed for 2–8 years. There was an immediate impression of improvement in ulnar drift, less extension deficit and improved flexion. Later, some deterioration occurred, although there were no fractures of the prostheses or synovitis. Good results also included an improvement in the patient's sense of well-being.

4. The Proximal Interphalangeal Joint

Nalebuff EA **Swan-neck deformity** In: Lamb DW, Hooper G, Kuczynski K, eds. The practice of hand surgery. 2nd edn. Oxford: Blackwell Scientific Publications, 1989:554–561

Heywood AWB **Rheumatoid boutonnière deformity** In: Lamb DW, Hooper G, Kuczynski K, eds. The practice of hand surgery. 2nd edn. Oxford: Blackwell Scientific Publications, 1989:561–565

Deformities of the fingers are often multiple and complicated, especially in the severely diseased rheumatoid hand. It is suggested that surgical treatment in such cases is the realm of surgeons with special knowledge and training. In these circumstances, two references are presented for rapid knowledge. **Nalebuff** described four types of deformity and noted that this represents an imbalance of the flexor and extensor forces acting on the various digital joints. Treatment is discussed for each of the four types. **Heywood** noted that approximately 15% of rheumatoid patients developed a Boutonnière deformity in one or more fingers. The basic pathology is erosion and stretching of the middle extensor slip at its insertion. Possible treatment methods are outlined for the three stages of this deformity.

5. The Thumb

Stanley (1988) JK **Surgical management of the rheumatoid wrist and hand. The surgery of the thumb.** In: Beddow FH, ed. Surgical management of rheumatoid arthritis. London: Wright, 1988:102–106

Stanley JK, Smith EJ, Muirhead AG **Arthrodesis of the metacarpophalageal joint of the thumb: a review of 42 cases** J Hand Surg [Br] 1989;14B:291–293

Stanley (1988) illustrated the types of deformity which occur in the thumb, previously classified by Nalebuff. Arthrodesis of the metacarpophalangeal joint constitutes one of the most rewarding surgical procedures that can be performed in the rheumatoid patient. **Stanley** (1989) described the results in 42 cases. The Omer chevron type of fusion was preferred and the joint fixed in flexion.

Tumours

Mankin HJ **Principles of diagnosis and management of tumours of the hand** Hand Clin 1987;3:2:185–195

Rosenberg AE, Schiller AL **Soft-tissue sarcomas of the hand** Hand Clin 1987;3:2:247–261

Louis DS **Peripheral nerve tumours in the upper extremity** Hand Clin 1987;3:2:311–318

Roberts PH, Price CHG **Chondrosarcoma of the bones of the hand** J Bone Joint Surg [Br] 1977;59B:213–221

Mankin stressed the development of a method of staging in the diagnosis and treatment of tumours, and its application to the hand. Metastatic carcinoma, lymphoma and myeloma are rarely encountered in the hand. Most primary bone tumours are benign. The most common bone tumours are enchondromas and osteocartilaginous exostoses. The third most common site for giant-cell tumours is the distal radius. Epithelioid sarcoma, synovioma and clear-cell sarcoma are common, and generally highly malignant. **Rosenberg** noted that soft-tissue sarcomas of the hand frequently have misleading clinical presentations, resulting in inappropriate therapy; they may have a prolonged clinical course with a high incidence of lymphatic spread. An ill-chosen biopsy site may necessitate more drastic surgery than originally required. **Louis** provided a useful reference for the treatment of peripheral nerve tumours in the upper extremity. **Roberts** reported a study of 19 rare aggressive cartilage tumours in the bones of the hand, from the Bristol Bone Tumour Registry.

Section 4

The Spine

The Neck

Cervical Disc and Degenerative Disease

Pathogenesis

Lestini WF, Wiesel SW **The pathogenesis of cervical spondylosis** Clin Orthop 1989;239:69–93

Lestini discussed the pathogenesis of both spondylotic radiculopathy and myelopathy. The two syndromes are distinct, yet they may overlap. The morbid anatomy, symptoms and nerve-root patterns are related. The importance of narrowing of both the foramina and the AP diameter of the cervical canal is stressed.

Radiology

Pelz DM, Fox AJ **Radiologic investigation In : Mini symposium: cervical disc and degenerative disease** Curr Orthop 1990;4:1:9–14

Pelz reviewed the value of the various radiological techniques available for screening and diagnosis. The role of MRI as a screening technique in cervical spondylosis remains controversial, particularly as demonstration of degenerative changes may have no relation to clinical symptoms. Nevertheless, myelography is gradually being replaced by MRI for patients with radiculopathy or myelopathy. The low inherent contrast has limited the usefulness of CT as a non-invasive technique.

Natural History

La Rocca H **Cervical spondylotic myelopathy: natural history** Spine 1988; 13:854–855

La Rocca discussed the variety of clinical courses of cervical spondylotic myelopathy. The most common pattern of progression is one of a series of episodes of new symptoms and signs. Sensory and sphincter changes tend to be transient. In introducing a symposium on cervical spondylotic myelopathy in the same journal (*Spine* 1988) White considered this subject to be the most common cause of spinal dysfunction in patients over 55 and the disease is probably "under-studied, under-diagnosed and under-treated".

Surgical Treatment

Herkowitz HN **The surgical management of cervical spondylotic radiculopathy and myelopathy** Clin Orthop 1989;239:94–108

Hukuda S, Mochizuki T, Ogata M, Shichikawa K, Shimomura Y **Operations for cervical spondylotic myelopathy: a comparison of the results of anterior and posterior procedures** J Bone Joint Surg [Br] 1985;67B:609–615

Hirabayashi K, Satomi K **Operative procedure and results of expansive open-door laminoplasty** Spine 1988;13:870–876

Herkowitz debated surgical treatment. Anterior discectomy and fusion was preferred for one- or two-level spondylotic radiculopathy. For the treatment of more extensive disease, the alternative is open-door laminoplasty, which is indicated particularly in developmental stenosis or failed anterior fusion. **Hukuda** described experience over 19 years with operations on 269 patients for myelopathy. The results of posterior operations were better than anterior for patients with more advanced myelopathies. Brachialgia, cord syndromes and central cord syndromes had a satisfactory outcome with anterior operations. The type of anterior or posterior operation made no difference. Patients with a short duration of symptoms fared better. **Hirabayashi** discussed the operative procedure, indications and results of open-door laminoplasty. Over 90 operations had been performed since the procedure was devised by the author in 1977. This procedure is considered to be superior to ordinary laminectomy; it prevents postoperative malalignment and reduces instability of the cervical spine.

Torticollis

Clinical Reviews

MacDonald D **Sternomastoid tumour and muscular torticollis** J Bone Joint Surg [Br] 1969;51B:432–443

Ferkel RD, Westin GW, Dawson EG, Oppenheim WL **Muscular torticollis: a modified surgical approach** J Bone Joint Surg [Am] 1983;65A:894–900

Ippolito E, Tudisco C, Massobrio M **Long-term results of open sternocleidomastoid tenotomy for idiopathic muscular torticollis** J Bone Joint Surg [Am] 1985;67A:30–38

Phillips WA, Hensinger RN **The management of rotatory atlantoaxial subluxation in children** J Bone Joint Surg [Am] 1989; 71A:664–668

MacDonald studied 50 patients presenting with a sternomastoid tumour and 52 who presented with a muscular torticollis. Only 1 in 7 patients with a tumour proceeded to muscular torticollis. The treatment by open division of the contracture is described. The operation will cure the principal deformity but not the facial asymmetry even if performed in the early years of life. **Ferkel** described a bipolar release and Z-plasty performed either when conservative treatment had failed, or in older children who had had other operations. **Ippolito** evaluated 67 patients who had undergone an open tenotomy of the origin of the sternomastoid muscle 15 years previously. The best results occurred in those who were operated on early between the ages of 5 months and 6 years. **Phillips** debated the problems of diagnosis and treatment of 23 children with torticollis secondary to rotatory atlantoaxial subluxation. Some presented with a history of minor trauma, others had suffered a recent respiratory infection. With a short history, the subluxation may reduce spontaneously or with traction. A few eventually needed a posterior atlantoaxial arthrodesis.

Rheumatoid Arthritis

Natural History

Pellicci PM, Ranawat CS, Tsairis P, Bryan WJ **A prospective study of the progression of rheumatoid arthritis of the cervical spine** J Bone Joint Surg [Am] 1981;63A:342–350

Lipson SJ **Rheumatoid arthritis in the cervical spine** Clin Orthop 1989;239: 121–127

Pellicci described a prospective study of the progression of rheumatoid arthritis in 106 patients. At the beginning of the study 43% of the patients had radiographic evidence of rheumatoid involvement of the cervical spine. Involvement at different levels is discussed, including atlantoaxial subluxation. Pain, neural involvement and radiographic abnormalities were progressive but radiographic deterioration was a more prominent feature than progressive neural dysfunction. Eighty-one per cent of the patients had radiographic deterioration whereas only 36% had progressive neural abnormality. The results of this study suggest that about 10% of patients with evidence of rheumatoid disease risk deterioration to a level requiring surgery. **Lipson** summarised knowledge of the pathology, natural history and surgical management. Subluxations are common, neurological problems less so. Once myelopathy is established, the natural history is poor. Neurological deterioration and pain are indications for surgery.

Surgical Treatment

Zoma A, Sturrock RD, Fisher WD, Freeman PA, Hamblen DL **Surgical stabilisation of the rheumatoid cervical spine: a review of indications and results** J Bone Joint Surg [Br] 1987;69B:8–12

Heywood AWB, Learmonth ID, Thomas M **Cervical spine instability in rheumatoid arthritis** J Bone Joint Surg [Br] 1988;70B:702–707

Wertheim SB, Bohlman HH **Occipitocervical fusion: indications, technique and long-term results in 13 patients** J Bone Joint Surg [Am] 1987;69A: 833–836

Santavirta S, Slatis P, Kankaanpaa U, Sandelin J, Laasonen E **Treatment of the cervical spine in rheumatoid arthritis** J Bone Joint Surg [Am] 1988;70A: 658–667

Clark CR, Goetz DD, Menezes AH **Arthrodesis of the cervical spine in rheumatoid arthritis** J Bone Joint Surg 1989;71A:381–392

Bonney G, Williams JPR **Transoral approach to the upper cervical spine: a report of 16 cases** J Bone Joint Surg [Br] 1985;67B:691–698

The surgical management of the rheumatoid cervical spine is controversial. There have been several large studies published on this subject recently. **Zoma** reviewed the indications and results of surgical stabilisation in 32 patients. The results were sometimes discouraging. Pain and radiographic instability without neurological deficit rarely required operation, but for progressive neurological impairment, surgery may be the only solution despite its hazards and disappointments. **Heywood** discussed the results of 30 fusion operations for cervical spine instability. Neurological compromise in an unstable but mobile rheumatoid cervical spine can usually be brought to remission by immobilisation alone; decompressive procedures were unnecessary in the first instance. **Wertheim** described a technique for occipitocervical fusion which had been performed in 13 patients. The indications for surgery were instability, neurological deficit or intractable pain. This type of arthrodesis should be undertaken before severe myelopathy occurs in patients who have instability of the cervical spine. **Santavirta** discussed experience with 34 patients, some of whom were treated operatively and some non-operatively. It was concluded that fusion of an unstable spine can relieve pain and prevent further impairment of function, but it will improve only slightly any existing neurological deficiency. Conservative treatment does not always prevent pain and it does not prevent progression of existing subluxations. **Clark** stressed the difficult challenge of treatment. When treated by arthrodesis, some of these patients are at risk of dying in the early postoperative period. Because of the likelihood of progressive instability, arthrodesis should be considered when there is evidence of major instability. Pseudarthrosis remains a problem and progression of instability to a higher level above the fusion is not uncommon. Evidence of an impending neurological deficit is an indication for early operation. The paper by **Bonney** has been included as a rapid reference to the subject of transoral approach to the upper cervical spine.

Down's Syndrome

Clinical Reviews

Burke SW, French HG, Roberts JM, Johnston CE, Whitecloud TS, Edmonds JO **Chronic atlantoaxial instability in Down syndrome** J Bone Joint Surg [Am] 1985;67A:1356–1360

Pueschel SM, Scola FH **Atlantoaxial instability in individuals with Down syndrome: epidemiologic, radiographic and clinical studies** Pediatrics 1987;80:555–560

Davidson RG **Atlantoaxial instability in individuals with Down syndrome: a fresk look at the evidence** Pediatrics 1988;81:857–865

Burke discussed the incidence of atlantoaxial instability in the radiographs of 32 patients. The condition is rare and occurs more commonly in boys over 10 years of age. **Pueschel** examined 404 patients. More than 85% had no evidence of instability and could participate in all sports activities. Thirteen per cent had asymptomatic instability and precautions had to be taken with this group of children. Surgical correction is necessary in 1%–2% who have symptomatic instability in order to prevent further spinal cord injury. **Davidson** debated the wisdom of these patients taking part in sports training and athletic competition. He concluded that there is no evidence to indicate that instability constitutes predisposition to dislocation. Some 500 000 individuals with this syndrome have participated in competitive sports with no reported cases of dislocation. These patients should not be excluded from sports but they should be examined to exclude abnormal neurological findings.

Lumbar Disc Disorders

Applied Anatomy

Crock HV **Normal and pathological anatomy of the lumbar spinal nerve root canals** J Bone Joint Surg [Br] 1981;63B:487–490

Postacchini F, Urso S, Ferro L **Lumbosacral nerve-root anomalies** J Bone Joint Surg [Am] 1982;64A:721–729

Crock presented a description of the normal anatomy of the lumbar spinal nerve root canals and the intervertebral foramen. The pathological anatomy was illustrated with particular reference to stenosis of the nerve root canals. **Postacchini** found 46 anomalous nerve roots in a series of over 2000 patients investigated by water-soluble radiculography. Five types were described. The nerve roots emerged either more cranially (type I) or more caudally (type II) or sometimes through closely adherent openings (type III). The anomalies were usually unilateral, and symptoms and signs of nerve root compression were often severe.

Pathogenesis

Farfan HF, Cossette JW, Robertson GH, Wells RV, Kraus H **The effects of torsion on the lumbar intervertebral joints: the role of torsion in the production of disc degeneration** J Bone Joint Surg [Am] 1979;52A:468–497

Yasuma T, Makino E, Saito S, Inui M **Histological development of intervertebral disc herniation** J Bone Joint Surg [Am] 1986;68A:1066–1072

Farfan presented evidence, based on a study of necropsy specimens, that torsional stresses as encountered in daily activity play a major role in initiating degeneration of the intervertebral discs. A degenerate disc is less able to resist rotation. Chronic rotation forces can produce microfractures in the lamina and further degeneration. **Yasuma** studied 257 intervertebral discs at autopsy and material from 441 operations for herniation of a disc. He described two types of protrusion: one the pulposus, the other an annular protrusion without involvement of the nucleus pulposus.

Epidemiology

Frymoyer JW, Newberg A, Pope MH, Wilder DG, Clements J, MacPherson B **Spine radiographs in patients with low back pain: in epidemiological study in men** J Bone Joint Surg [Am] 1984;66A:1048–1055

Frymoyer performed a random study of 292 adult males to determine the value of radiographic studies in the assessment of low back pain. One-third had never had low back pain, 45% had had moderate pain and 22% had experienced severe pain. There was an increased incidence of low back pain where there were traction spurs or disc space narrowing between the 4th and 5th lumbar vertebrae, but plain radiography was of little use in determining the causes of low back pain in men between the ages of 18 and 55.

Clinical Studies – Low Back Pain

Nachemson AL **Advances in low back pain** Clin Orthop 1985;200:266–273

Frymoyer JW **Medical progress in back pain and sciatica** N Engl J Med 1988;318:291–300

Waddell G, McCulloch JA, Kummel E, Venner RM **Non-organic physical signs in low back pain** Spine 1980;5:117–125

Waddell G, Main CJ, Morris EW, Di Paola M, Gray ICM **Chronic low back pain, psychological distress and illness behaviour** Spine 1984;9:209–213

Fredrickson BE, Trief PM, Van Beveren P, Yuan HA, Baum G **Rehabilitation of the patient with chronic back pain: a search for outcome predictors** Spine 1988;13:351–353

Nachemson stressed the good natural history of low back pain. Only 10% suffer disabling pain for more than 6 weeks. The use of the various types of treatment for low back pain and sciatica are debated. Repeated surgery should be avoided if at all possible. **Frymoyer** discussed the epidemiology, natural history and treatment of acute low back pain, subacute pain and sciatica with chronic pain. The contributions by **Waddell** are well recognised. In 1980, non-organic physical signs were described, such as tenderness, inappropriate responses and over-reaction; they are distinguishable from the signs of pathology and can be used as a clinical screen to identify patients who require more detailed psychological assessment. In 1984, **Waddell** described methods of assessment of distress and illness behaviour in chronic low back pain. **Fredrickson** attempted to identify the outcome in patients admitted to a rehabilitation programme for chronic low back pain. Patients over the age of 50 returned to work with much less frequency than those younger than 50. Psychological information from the MMPI was of no value. This paper has been included since it demonstrates the difficulty in prediction of outcome in the case of an individual patient.

Radiological Investigation

Bell GR, Rothman RH, Booth RE, Cuckler JM, Garfin S, Herkowitz H, Simeone FA, Dolinskas C, Han SS **A study of computer-assisted tomography. II. Comparison of metrizamide myelography and computed tomography in the diagnosis of herniated lumbar disc and spinal stenosis** Spine 1984;9: 552–556

Boden SD, Davis DO, Dina TS, Patronas NJ, Wiesel SW **Abnormal magnetic resonance scans of the lumbar spine in asymptomatic subjects: a prospective investigation** J Bone Joint Surg [Am] 1990;72A:403–408

Szypryt EP, Twining P, Wilde GP, Mulholland RC, Worthing BS **Diagnosis of lumbar disc protrusion: A comparison between magnetic resonance imaging and radiculography** J Bone Joint Surg [Br] 1988;70B:717–722

Colhoun E, McCall IW, Williams L, Cassar Pullicino VN **Provocation discography as a guide to planning operations on the spine** J Bone Joint Surg [Br] 1988;70B:267–271

Fraser RD, Osti OL, Vernon-Roberts B **Discitis after discography** J Bone Joint Surg [Br] 1987;69B:26–35

Hueftle MG, Modic MT, Ross JS, Masaryk TJ, Carter JR, Wilber RG, Bohlman HH, Steinbeg PM, Delamarter RB **Lumbar spine: postoperative MR imaging with GD-DTPAl** Radiology 1988;167:817–824

The precise value of myelography, discography and MRI is controversial. **Bell** considered myelography was more accurate than tomography in the diagnosis of both lumbar disc protrusion and spinal stenosis, and had the advantage of allowing examination at more levels. **Boden** performed MRI on individuals who had never had low back pain or sciatica. The findings were abnormal in about 57% of patients 60 years of age or older. Abnormalities on MRI must be strictly correlated with clinical presentation before operative treatment is contemplated. **Szypryt** compared the value of MRI and radiculograms in 42 consecutive patients. MRI predicted the correct diagnosis in 88%, radiculography in 75%. MRI is slightly better than radiculography in diagnosing lumbar disc protrusions. **Colhoun** attempted to define the role of discography in the investigation of patients with lumbar disease. The records of 195 patients were studied 2 years after a technically successful operation. Where discography had revealed disc disease and provoked symptoms, 89% derived benefit from operation. Conversely, operation was less successful where no provocation of symptoms occurred on discography. **Fraser** discussed the rare complication of discitis after discography. Discitis occurred in 2.7% of 222 patients. It was suggested that all cases were initiated by infection and that a very strict aseptic technique must be used for discography. **Hueftle** performed MRI with special techniques in 30 patients with "failed back surgery syndrome". The studies were highly accurate in separating epidural fibrosis from herniated disc.

THE SPINE

Treatment – Medical

Deyo RA, Diehl AK, Rosenthal M **Special article: how many days of bed rest for acute low back pain? A randomised clinical trial** N Engl J Med 1986;315: 17:1064–1070

Haldeman S **Spinal manipulative therapy: a status report** Clin Orthop 1983;179:63–70

Cuckler JM, Bernini PA, Wiesel SW, Booth RE, Rothman RH, Pickens GT **The use of epidural steroids in the treatment of lumbar radicular pain – a prospective randomised double-blind study** J Bone Joint Surg [Am] 1985; 67A:63–66

White AH, Derby R, Wynne G **Epidural injections for the diagnosis and treatment of low-back pain** Spine 1980;5:78–86

Frymoyer and **Nachemson** (see Clinical Studies) provided a general review on the principles of medical treatment of lumbar pain. **Deyo** noted that the optimum duration of bed rest for acute pain is uncertain. In a study of 203 patients with mechanical low back pain and without neurological deficit, one group was given 2 days of bed rest and the other 7 days. No difference was noted in the outcome. Data support a trend towards earlier mobilisation of patients with acute back pain. It was suggested that if widely applied, this policy might reduce costs for both patients and employers. **Haldeman** discussed the value of manipulation, both for diagnosis and treatment. Categories of manipulative treatment are discussed. The effectiveness of manipulation is greatest in patients who have acute lumbar pain and no leg pain or neurological deficit. Complications are rare but can be catastrophic. **Cuckler** compared patients treated with epidural injections either with steroids and procaine or saline and procaine. No statistical difference was observed between the two groups, in either an acute disc or with spinal stenosis. It was concluded that there was no evidence of clinical efficacy of epidural steroids in lumbar pain. **White** performed a prospective randomised double-blind trial of 304 consecutive patients. Whilst many had temporary relief, only 1.3% had no recurrence of symptoms within 2 years. It was concluded that epidural steroids could shorten the clinical course but did not produce a cure.

Treatment – Surgical

1. Review Articles

Eismont FJ, Currier B **Current concepts review: surgical management of lumbar intervertebral-disc disease** J Bone Joint Surg [Am] 1989;71A: 1266–1271

Porter RW, Hibbert CS, Wicks M **The spinal canal in symptomatic lumbar disc lesions** J Bone Joint Surg [Br] 1978;60B:485–487

Eismont noted that imaging techniques must be able to differentiate between sequestrated disc fragments and an extruded or prolapsed disc since this is critical when considering which treatment to perform. The criteria for standard discectomy, limited discectomy and microsurgical lumbar discectomy are stressed. The use of chemonucleolysis is critically assessed. The newer procedures have a learning curve and each has associated complications, but they shorten hospitalisation and may decrease postoperative convalescence. **Porter** measured by diagnostic ultrasound the oblique sagittal diameter of the lumbar spinal canal. Fifty-five per cent of patients with disabling disc symptoms had narrow canals of trefoil shape.

2. Central Disc Prolapse

Kostuik JP, Harrington I, Alexander D, Rand W, Evans D **Corda equina syndrome and lumbar disc herniation** J Bone Joint Surg [Am] 1986;68A: 386–391

Kostuik identified two modes of presentation in a study of 31 patients. The first was acute, with abrupt severe symptoms and signs and a poor prognosis for bladder function. The second was slower in onset, with symptoms prior to the onset of the cauda equina syndrome. All had sciatica, although this was not necessarily bilateral. There was no correlation between the urgency of decompression and the return of function, although early surgery was recommended. The well-recognised papers by Jennet and Scott are referred to in this article and together, these three contributions have important medicolegal connotations for the treatment of an acute central disc protrusion, particularly with bladder involvement.

3. Standard Discectomy

Weber H **Lumbar disc herniation. A controlled prospective study with 10 years' observation** Spine 1983;8:131–140

Spengler DM **Lumbar discectomy: results with limited disc excision and selective foraminotomy** Spine 1982;7:604–607

Hanley EN, Shapiro DE **The development of low-back pain after excision of a lumbar disc** J Bone Joint Surg [Am] 1989;71A:719–721

Weber compared the results of surgical and conservative treatment in patients with an uncertain indication for surgery. The operated patients showed better results both at 1 year and 4 years after surgery. **Spengler** considered limited disc excision to be a safe and effective method of treating selected patients. His data did not support concern over an increased incidence of recurrent disc herniation with this kind of operation; however, the surgeon must be prepared to perform a foraminotomy if the nerve root remains tight after disc excision. **Hanley** stressed the importance of disabling low back pain (14%) in a series of 120 consecutive patients who had been relieved of their sciatic pain. Narrowing of the disc space was almost always present but this did not correlate with the degree of pain.

4. Discectomy and Fusion

Frymoyer JW, Hanley E, Howe J, Kuhlmann D, Matteri R **Disc excision and spine fusion in the management of disc disease: a minimum 10 year follow-up** Spine 1978;3:1–6

White AH, Von Rongov P, Zucherman J, Heiden D **Lumbar laminectomy for herniated disc: a prospective controlled comparison with internal fixation fusion** Spine 1987;12:305–307

Two papers have been included which have addressed the debate as to the results of disc excision with and without spinal fusion. The conclusions were similar. **Frymoyer** analysed the results of surgery on 312 patients observed for 10 years; there was a remarkable similarity in the occupational status of those who underwent spinal fusion and those who did not. **White**, in a 10-year prospective study, compared the results in patients with and without immediate internal fixation after the disc excision. The addition of fixation did not increase the subjective or objective success rate and those with a fusion had a significantly longer mean time to return to work. It was concluded that a fusion is not necessary and gives less satisfactory results in simple laminectomy cases for herniated lumbar disc.

5. Microsurgical Lumbar Discectomy

Williams RW **Microlumbar discectomy: a 12-year statistical review** Spine 1986;11:851–852

Thomas AMC, Afshar F **The microsurgical treatment of lumbar disc protrusion: follow-up of 60 cases** J Bone Joint Surg [Br] 1987;69B:696–698

Williams described the "simple operative technique" of microlumbar discectomy in 1978. The operation was developed for patients with undisturbed lumbar anatomy with a soft disc herniation and no lumbar stenosis. The diagnosis was confirmed by CT scan. The principal features of the technique are described, stressing visualisation of the nerve root at all times and no curettement of the disc tissue. Results of surgery in 903 patients are described. Reoperation was necessary in 14%. Limitation of excessive physical activity was advised during the postoperative year. **Thomas** discussed the technique of this operation. Ninety-one per cent of patients had good or excellent results. CT scanning was not available when most of the patients in this series presented but all had a positive radiculogram. The use of the microscope is stressed. Some details of technique are different from those described by Williams.

6. Percutaneous Discectomy

Onik G, Helms CA, Ginnesberg L, Hoaglund FT, Morris J **Percutaneous lumbar discectomy using a new aspiration probe** AJR 1985;144:1137–1140

Hijikata S **Percutaneous nucleotomy: a new concept technique and 12 years' experience** Clin Orthop 1989;238:9–23

Percutaneous discectomy was designed to decompress mechanically a herniated disc through a posterolaterally inserted cannula. **Onik,** in 1985, described a relatively non-invasive means of disc decompression by the insertion of a specialised probe into the disc space and withdrawal of the disc by suction. The probe tip is round and blunt, and insertion is performed under local anaesthesia. A symposium on this subject was reported in 1989 (Clin Orthop 238). One paper from this symposium has been included by **Hijikata**. The procedure and experience is described and illustrated in detail.

7. Complications of Surgical Treatment: Vascular Injuries

Birkeland IW, Taylor TKF **Major vascular injuries in lumbar disc surgery** J Bone Joint Surg [Br] 1969;51B:4–19

Four cases of vascular injury during lumbar disc removal are reported and illustrated in detail. Although this paper was published in 1969, cases do still occur and the possibility of vascular injury should be kept in mind during laminectomy for disc prolapse – especially at the L4/5 level.

8. Complications of Surgical Treatment: Arachnoiditis

Ransford AO, Harries BJ **Localised arachnoiditis complicating lumbar disc lesions** J Bone Joint Surg [Br] 1972;54B:656–665

Hoyland JA, Freemont AJ, Denton J, Thomas AMC, McMillan JJ, Jayson MIV
Retained surgical swab debris in post-laminectomy arachnoiditis and peridural fibrosis J Bone Joint Surg [Br] 1988;70B:659–662

Ransford presented case reports of 5 patients suffering from arachnoiditis following disc operations. **Hoyland** observed that arachnoiditis may lead to intractable nerve root pain which is difficult to control. Twenty-six patients referred to a neurosurgical department were described. Dense connective tissue was found about the nerve roots. The possible aetiology and treatment of this difficult complication is debated.

Chemonucleolysis

McCulloch JA **Chemonucleolysis** J Bone Joint Surg [Br] 1977;59B:45–52

Wiltse LL **Chemonucleolysis in the treatment of lumbar disc disease** In: McKibbin B, ed. Recent advances in orthopaedics 4. 1983:103–108

Hall BB, McCulloch JA **Anaphylactic reactions following the intradiscal injection of chymopapain under local anaesthesia** J Bone Joint Surg [Am] 1983;65A:1215–1219

Gibson MJ, Buckley J, Mulholland RC, Worthington BS **The changes in the intervertebral disc after chemonucleolysis demonstrated by magnetic resonance imaging** J Bone Joint Surg [Br] 1986;68B:719–723

McCulloch described in 1977 the results of a prospective study of 480 patients treated by chemonucleolysis. Seventy per cent with a disc herniation had a favourable response. The most common failure was persistent back pain. The causes of poor results were discussed. In 1983, **Wiltse** reviewed the use of chemonucleolysis in the treatment of lumbar disc disease. The technique was described. **Wiltse** considered the procedure to be both safe and effective. In patients with definite neurological change in the form of reflex, motor or sensory disturbance, 74% had reverted to normal 1 year post-injection. An extradural disc is not a contraindication to treatment, but a sequestrated disc is. Anaphylaxis does occur but is rare and can be anticipated and safeguarded with the use of steroids. **Hall** described these reactions in an experience of over 4000 patients over 11 years. Fifteen occurred but 12 had subjective early warning signs. Hypotension requiring vigorous treatment was the life-threatening clinical manifestation of anaphylaxis. There were no deaths. Local anaesthesia is mandatory so that early warning by the patient may be given. **Eismont** (1989, see above) summarised the use of chemonucleolysis at the present time. The popularity of its use in the United States has decreased dramatically because of adverse effects, particularly the risk of neurological catastrophe, although the latter is very rare. **Gibson** showed a consistent pattern of gradual loss of signal from the nucleus pulposus after chemonucleolysis. MRI changes were produced analogous with premature gross disc degeneration.

Facet Arthritis

Eisenstein SM, Parry CR **The lumbar facet arthrosis syndrome: clinical presentation and articular surface changes** J Bone Joint Surg [Br] 1987;69B: 3–7

Jackson RP, Jacobs RR, Montesano PX **Facet joint injection in low back pain: a prospective statistical study** Spine 1988;13:966–971

Getty CJM, Johnson JR, Kirwan EO'G, Sullivan MF **Partial undercutting facetectomy for bony entrapment of the lumbar nerve root** J Bone Joint Surg [Br] 1981;63B:330–335

Three papers have been included which reflect growing interest in the facet joints as a cause of low back pain and sciatica. **Eisenstein** described a syndrome where disabling symptoms are associated with normal radiographs. Local spinal fusion relieved symptoms in certain patients. The excised facet joint showed cartilage necrosis but no osteophytes. It is suggested that facet arthrosis may be an important cause of severe back pain in young and middle-aged adults. **Jackson** reported the results of a prospective study on 390 patients with back pain and no neurological signs who had facet joint injections. Facet joint arthrograms were performed on all prior to the injection. Initial pain relief occurred in only 29%. Greatest pain relief occurred with lumbar extension and rotation. Facet joints were not considered the source of low back pain in the majority of these patients. **Getty** described the results in 78 patients who had been operated on for bony entrapment of a lumbar nerve root. Many had previously undergone spinal operations. Pain in the leg was the predominant symptom. The principal factor in the aetiology was degenerative change in the posterior facet joints. Most patients were satisfied with lasting pain relief.

Lumbar Instability

Stokes IAF, Frymoyer JW **Segmental motion and instability** Spine 1987;12: 688–691

Dove J **Internal fixation of the lumbar spine: the Hartshill rectangle** Clin Orthop 1986;203:135–140

Symptoms and signs of lumbar instability have remained poorly defined and controversial. **Stokes** described the presentation and radiological features of 78 patients categorised as having degenerate instability. There was a tendency towards abnormal intersegmental motion of the lumbosacral spine but flexion–extension biplanar radiographs were not useful in the diagnosis of lumbar instability. The paper helps to summarise this difficult problem and is a useful recent reference. **Dove** described the Hartshill rectangle fixation, which is a modification of the Luque system of segmental spinal instrumentation. The technique provides good rotational stability and is described in detail.

Lumbar Disc Prolapse in Adolescence

Taylor TKF **Lumbar disc prolapse in adolescence.** In: Dickson RA, ed. Spinal surgery: science and practice. London: Butterworths, 1990:178–186

Gibson MJ, Szypryt EP, Buckley JH, Worthington BS, Mulholland RC **Magnetic resonance imaging of adolescent disc herniation** J Bone Joint Surg [Br] 1987; 69B:699–703

Lorenz M, McCulloch J **Chemonucleolysis for herniated nucleus pulposus in adolescents** J Bone Joint Surg [Am] 1985;67A:1402–1404

Taylor stressed the characteristic features of the presentation, with marked stiffness and pain and usually absent neurological signs. Treatment is controversial. Discectomy produced good immediate symptomatic relief but physical signs were slow to resolve. Experience with 35 cases had led to a more conservative approach, since at surgery sometimes a swollen nerve root was found without a large disc prolapse. **Gibson** discussed advances in diagnosis with the use of magnetic resonance imaging. In all patients a symptomatic disc produced an abnormal signal and in most a herniated fragment of nucleus pulposus was identified. **Lorenz** summarised the results of treatment of 55 adolescents with chemonucleolysis. This method of treatment was an effective and safe alternative to surgical excision in adolescents. It was only considered after the patient had failed to respond to conservative management. However, chemonucleolysis commonly produced increased back pain after injection, and it did not relieve the symptoms in approximately 20%. These patients all subsequently had surgical excision.

Spondylolisthesis

The Classic

Wiltse LL, Newman PH, MacNab I **Classification of spondylolysis and spondylolisthesis** Clin Orthop 1976,117:23–29

In 1976, **Wiltse, Newman** and **MacNab** described a working classification derived from previous ones published by the individual authors, which is in standard use today. There were five groups: I dysplastic, II isthmic, III degenerative, IV traumatic and V pathological. The salient features of the disorder were presented, based on both aetiological and anatomical factors.

Aetiology

Wiltse LL, Widell EH, Jackson DW **Fatigue fracture: the basic lesion in isthmic spondylolisthesis** J Bone Joint Surg [Am] 1975;57A:17–22

Wynne-Davies R, Scott JHS **Inheritance and spondylolisthesis: a radiographic family survey** J Bone Joint Surg [Br] 1979;61B:301–305

The cause of the isthmic type has been much debated. **Wiltse** considered the defect in the pars interarticularis was most often the result of repeated trauma, stress and factors other than acute fracture. The clinician should be aware of fatigue fracture and its consequences, sometimes with a marked slip. **Wynne-Davies** debated in detail the significance of inheritance in spondylolisthesis based on a study of the relatives of 47 patients. The 1 in 3 risk of spondylolysis to near relatives of patients with the dysplastic form of the condition was emphasised, in order that the deformity could be recognised at an early age.

Natural History

Fredrickson BE, Baker D, McHolick WJ, Yuan HA, Lubicky JP **The natural history of spondylolysis and spondylolisthesis** J Bone Joint Surg [Am] 1984; 66A:699–707

The natural history of isthmic spondylolisthesis has been debated for many years but never fully documented. **Fredrickson** examined the incidence of spondylolysis in a prospective study of 500 unselected first-grade children. At the age of 6 years it was 4.4%, and this increased to 6% in adulthood. Progression of a slip was unlikely after adolescence and the slip was never symptomatic in the population studied. A child with asymptomatic spondylolysis or spondylolisthesis can be permitted to enjoy a normal childhood without restriction of activities or fear of progressive listhesis.

Radiology

McAfee PC, Yuan HA **Computed tomography in spondylolisthesis** Clin Orthop 1982;166:62–71

Grenier N, Kressel HY, Schiebler ML, Grossman RI **Isthmic spondylolysis of the lumbar spine: MR imaging at 1.5 T1** Radiology 1989;170:489–493

McAfee studied the main benefits of computed tomography in 31 patients with all types of spondylolisthesis. It was most useful in patients with neurological symptoms and usually demonstrated the site of neural encroachment. Neurological findings in this condition can be due to a multitude of anatomical abnormalities and should not be simply attributed to a herniated nucleus pulposus at the site of the slip. **Grenier** compared the appearance on magnetic resonance images of the normal pars interarticularis with that of the pars with spondylolysis. MRI poorly delineated bone fragments around the defect but revealed complications such as herniation of the disc above.

Surgery

Wiltse LL, Jackson DW **Treatment of spondylolisthesis and spondylolysis in children** Clin Orthop 1976;117:92–100

Harris IE, Weinstein SL **Long-term follow-up of patients with Grade III and IV spondylolisthesis: treatment with and without posterior fusion** J Bone Surg [Am] 1987;69A:960–969

Pedersen AK, Hagen R **Spondylolysis and spondylolisthesis: treatment by internal fixation and bone grafting of the defect** J Bone Joint Surg [Am] 1988; 70A:15–24

Bradford DS, Gotfried Y **Staged salvage reconstruction of Grade IV and V spondylolisthesis** J Bone Joint Surg [Am] 1987;69A:191–202

Seitsalo S, Osterman K, Hyvarinen H, Schlenzka D, Poussa M **Severe spondylolisthesis in children and adolescents: a long term review of fusion in situ** J Bone Joint Surg [Br] 1990;72B:259–265

Wiltse considered that most children with spondylolisthesis never developed significant symptoms, and even in those who did, the vast majority could be treated without surgery. If symptoms persist, or if further displacement is occurring, a one-level spinal fusion was recommended. A precise technique was described and illustrated (previously described in 1968). Solid fusion can always be obtained and will prevent further slip. **Harris** compared the long-term results of patients with severe spondylolisthesis with and without posterior fusion. In situ arthrodesis provided acceptable results at an average 20-year follow-up; the patients were less symptomatic and less restricted in their activities than were the nonoperatively treated patients. The degree of slip at the time of fusion did not influence the result. **Pedersen** narrated experience with the Buck method for bone grafting and screw fixation of the defect of the pars interarticularis in 18 patients with mild displacement. A satisfactory result was obtained in 83%. The procedure was stated to be less formidable than the posterolateral arthrodesis with less surgical dissection required. It should be limited to younger adults without secondary degenerative changes. **Bradford** described special experience with 16 patients with progression of deformity after surgery, sometimes with incapacitating pain. It was concluded that staged reconstructive surgery was feasible as a salvage procedure; these operations carried a greater risk than the more established technique of fusion in situ, but the benefits outweighed the risks. **Seitsalo** studied the result of treatment of 87 adolescents observed for 14 years. All had a fusion operation performed in situ, the majority being posterior, some posterolateral and a few anterior. There were no major complications, although a significant number required reoperation for nonunion. One in four had 10% or more progression of the slip after fusion. Fusion was considered a safe operation with good long-term results, although increase of lumbosacral kyphosis may cause problems outside the area of fusion.

Review Article

Hensinger RN **Current concepts review: spondylolysis and spondylolisthesis in children and adolescents** J Bone Joint Surg [Am] 1989;71A:1098–1107

A comprehensive recent review article has been written by **Hensinger**. There is detailed discussion on the value of bone scans and the risk factors that are important in assessment of the untreated patient with symptomatic spondylolisthesis. The results of in situ arthrodesis are excellent, even after 20 years of follow-up.

Spinal Stenosis

Review Article

Spengler DM **Current concepts review: degenerative stenosis of the lumbar spine** J Bone Joint Surg [Am] 1987;69A:305–308

Spengler provided a concise review of this subject. The insidious onset in older patients was stressed, with a variable pattern of symptoms but especially with changes in position. There were few findings on physical examination and signs of tension on the sciatic nerve were found only occasionally. Myelography is both valuable and essential. With careful selection, decompression results in a good outcome in 85%.

Pathology and Diagnosis

Naylor A **Factors in the development of the spinal stenosis syndrome** J Bone Joint Surg [Br] 1979;61B:306–309

Bolender NF, Schonstrom NSR, Spengler DM **Role of computed tomography and myelography in the diagnosis of central spinal stenosis** J Bone Joint Surg [Am] 1985;67A:240–246

Naylor discussed factors in the development of this syndrome, stressing the narrowing of the canal increased by posterolateral bulging of the annulus fibrosus. Diagrams representing axial tomograms are shown, both of the normal and abnormal spine. To relieve symptoms, the nerve roots must be decompressed by full lateral decompression, with partial or total facetectomy if necessary. **Bolender** debated the value of computed tomography and myelography in 24 patients who underwent surgery. Computed tomography was much less reliable in providing a correct diagnosis than myelography, the latter being accurate in 83%. A narrow dural sac demonstrated by either method indicated central spinal stenosis.

Treatment

Wiltse LL, Kirkaldy-Willis H, McIvor GWD **The treatment of spinal stenosis** Clin Orthop 1976;115:83–91

Hall S, Bartleson JD, Onofrio BM, Baker HL, Okazaki H, O'Duffy JD **Lumbar spinal stenosis: clinical features, diagnostic procedures and the results of surgical treatment in 68 patients** Ann Intern Med 1985;103:271–275

In a symposium on the subject, **Wiltse** discussed treatment. The principles of surgery were outlined and illustrated, including the need for release of the spinal nerve trapped in the lateral recess and sometimes more laterally. Rarely, massive posterior decompression may be necessary. **Hall** reviewed the clinical features and results of treatment in 68 patients where the diagnosis was confirmed, and follow-up was for a minimum of 2.5 years. The most common presenting symptom was pseudo-claudication, which was present in 94% and included pain, numbness and weakness. Symptoms were usually bilateral, worse on walking, eased by sitting. All had extensive surgery particularly at the L2/3/4 levels, and 30% had stenosis at several levels. Four years after surgery, 84% reported that surgery had yielded good to excellent results. The precise pathogenesis remains uncertain and it may be a mechanical abnormality, since EMGs showed multiple radiculopathies.

Scoliosis

Congenital Scoliosis

McMaster MJ, Ohtsuka K **The natural history of congenital scoliosis: a study of 251 patients** J Bone Joint Surg [Am] 1982;64A:1128–1147

Winter RB, Moe JH, Lonstein JE **Posterior spinal arthrodesis for congenital scoliosis: an analysis of the cases of 290 patients, 5–19 years old** J Bone Joint Surg [Am] 1984;66A:1188–1197

Andrew T, Piggott H **Growth arrest for progressive scoliosis: combined anterior and posterior fusion of the convexity** J Bone Joint Surg [Br] 1985; 67B:193–197

In a comprehensive study, **McMaster** presented the variable prognosis for a patient with this condition. Some are first seen with small curves which deteriorate minimally, others with large curves that deteriorate rapidly and cause extreme deformity. The prognosis for untreated curves after the age of 10 years generally becomes more unfavourable. Ninety per cent of the curves could be classified into five groups. The ultimate severity of the curve depended on the type of anomaly and the site where it occurred. The prognosis was worst with unilateral unsegmented bars associated with contralateral hemivertebra. If seen initially in the first 2 years of life or at puberty, there was a bad prognosis. A curve that is at risk for progression can be recognised. **Winter** analysed the results of posterior fusion with or without Harrington instrumentation. The most common problem was bending of the fusion mass in growing children, which occurred in 14%. The use of the Harrington instruments allowed slightly better correction; operation should be performed early before severe deformity develops. On a small number of patients, **Andrew** discussed the use of epiphysiodesis combined with posterior fusion, both on the convex side. Progressive correction of the curve with growth was demonstrated. Full assessment must await skeletal maturity of these patients.

Infantile Scoliosis

Dickson RA **Early-onset idiopathic scoliosis** In: Review article: conservative treatment for idiopathic scoliosis J Bone Joint Surg [Br] 1985;67B:176–181

McMaster MJ **Infantile idiopathic scoliosis: can it be prevented?** J Bone Joint Surg [Br] 1983;65B:612–617

Thompson SK, Bentley G **Prognosis in infantile idiopathic scoliosis** J Bone Joint Surg [Br] 1980;62B:151–154

McMaster MJ, MacNicol MF **The management of progressive infantile idiopathic scoliosis** J Bone Joint Surg [Br] 1979;61B:36–42

Dickson summarised the natural history and treatment of infantile scoliosis. Three types were recognised, progressive, static and resolving. In the most serious, progression occurs in the hypotonic low-weight baby; there is some evidence that this condition can be treated conservatively. **McMaster** (1983), reported that the incidence of these infantile curves has rapidly declined and that the condition is now rare; it was concluded that infantile scoliosis is a preventable deformity and that this decline is due to prone lying in the cot. **Thompson** illustrated the method of measurement of infantile scoliosis by assessment of the rib vertebrae angle difference as described by Mehta. The prognosis was difficult to establish before the age of 5 years. If a scoliosis of 50° or more was present before the age of 4, it always progressed. Factors influencing the prognosis were discussed. **McMaster** debated the long term management. The aim was to recognise the progressive curve early, start immediate conservative treatment and fuse at the age of 10. The postoperative correction was 40% of the curve which was present in the child before treatment. Spinal fusion was associated with a moderate loss in correction due to bending of the fusion mass. Double structural curves were treated only in a brace. This provided less satisfactory control of these curves, but because of the minimal cosmetic deformity, extensive spinal fusion was avoided.

Screening

Torell G, Nordwall A, Nachemson A **The changing pattern of scoliosis treatment due to effective screening** J Bone Joint Surg [Am] 1981;63A: 337–341

Lonstein JE, Bjorklund S, Wanninger MH, Nelson RP **Voluntary school screening for scoliosis in Minnesota** J Bone Joint Surg [Am] 1982;64A: 481–488

Renshaw TS **Screening school children for scoliosis** Clin Orthop 1988;229: 26–33

The effects of a 10-year programme for early detection and treatment of idiopathic scoliosis in a stable population in Sweden were assessed by **Torell**. Seven hundred and twenty-five patients with a scoliosis of more than 20° were followed. The percentage of patients requiring operation each year decreased as did the number of severe cases detected. Screening was associated with a three-fold increase in the number of patients treated. **Lonstein** reviewed experience of a voluntary statewide school screening programme for scoliosis in Minnesota. Screening had been in operation for 8 years. Screening of a quarter of a million yearly led to a diagnosis of scoliosis in 1.2%. The effectiveness of the programme was seen in a decrease in the number of adolescents requiring surgical treatment. Screening was efficient and cost-effective. **Renshaw** noted that the advantages of screening are now recognised but costs are not inconsequential, and vast numbers of small non-progressive curves are discovered and followed. Continuing controversies include the age for screening, the criteria for referral for treatment and the efficacy of nonoperative treatment.

Late-Onset Idiopathic Scoliosis

Pathology

Dickson RA, Lawton JO, Archer IA, Butt WP **The pathogenesis of idiopathic scoliosis: biplanar spinal asymmetry** J Bone Joint Surg [Br] 1984;66B:8–15

The pathology of scoliosis remains difficult to understand and controversial. **Dickson** explored the pathology of idiopathic scoliosis in a clinical, cadaveric and radiological study. The basic feature is flattening or reversal of the normal thoracic kyphosis at the apex of the scoliosis, which leads to rotational instability. Rotation of the vertebrae then occurs with growth, which leads to the secondary deformity. The lateral profile of the spine is the key to the understanding of progressive idiopathic deformity.

Natural History

Weinstein SL, Zavala DC, Ponseti IV **Idiopathic scoliosis: long-term follow-up and prognosis in untreated patients** J Bone Joint Surg [Am] 1981;63A: 702–712

Weinstein SL, Ponseti IV **Curve progression in idiopathic scoliosis** J Bone Joint Surg [Am] 1983;65A:447–455

Weinstein described the results of a long-term follow-up (average 40 years) of 194 patients with untreated adolescent scoliosis. Backache was more common than in the general public but never disabling. The backache was unrelated to the presence of osteoarthritic changes. Pulmonary function was affected only in patients with thoracic curves. In a further study, **Weinstein** found that 68% of the curves progressed after skeletal maturity. In general, curves that were less than 30° at maturity tended not to progress regardless of curve pattern. Conversely, in curves of 50°–75°, especially thoracic progression was marked.

Conservative Treatment

Dickson RA **Conservative treatment for idiopathic scoliosis** J Bone Joint Surg [Br] 1985;67B:176–181

Edgar MA **Editorial: to brace or not to brace?** J Bone Joint Surg [Br] 1985; 67B:173–174

Emans JB, Kaelin A, Bancel P, Hall JE, Miller ME **The Boston bracing system for idiopathic scoliosis: follow-up results in 295 patients** Spine 1986;11:8: 792–801

Dickson reviewed the value of conservative treatment, including bracing, cast management and electrical stimulation. In late-onset idiopathic scoliosis, the larger the deformity, the greater the likelihood of social and psychological complications. With the advent of screening, the need for treatment has become less. Dickson considered that there was no evidence that Milwaukee brace treatment altered the course of the scoliosis. The use of electrical stimulation stemmed from a belief that there was a neuromuscular basis to the deformity; this is unlikely and there is no evidence that correction followed electrical stimulation. In an editorial, **Edgar** posed the fundamental question: is the death knell beginning to sound for brace treatment? He concluded that the literature is equivocal. There is a trend away from bracing but there is still a place for this method of treatment, especially for the progressive scoliosis with a 30°–40° curve. The need for a prospective controlled trial was considered to be paramount. **Emans** reviewed experience with 295 patients treated with the Boston bracing system. Indications for its use, and loss of correction after bracing, were discussed. Control or net correction of idiopathic scoliosis was achieved in 80%. Factors which affect the outcome of bracing were discussed.

Surgical Treatment

1. Review Article

Kostuik JP **Current concepts review: operative treatment of idiopathic scoliosis** J Bone Joint Surg [Am] 1990;72A:1108–1113

Operative intervention remains the definitive form of treatment. The use of sublaminar wires, anterior instrumentation and posterior derotation with Cotrel–Dubousset instrumentation have improved operative results, but they have increased the risk of neurological damage. The major indication for operation in an adolescent or young adult is progression of the curve to more than 45°–50°. Twenty-five per cent of patients operated on are adults, with pain as the primary reason for treatment. For the single thoracic curve, Cotrel–Dubousset instrumentation appears to be the method of choice. The disadvantages of this type of instrumentation are debated.

2. Selection of Levels of Fusion

King HA, Moe JH, Bradford DS, Winter RB **The selection of fusion levels in thoracic idiopathic scoliosis** J Bone Joint Surg [Am] 1983;65A:1302–1313

King discussed the selection of fusion level in thoracic scoliosis. A study of 405 patients was presented. Careful preoperative curve evaluation was essential to decide the exact levels of fusion. Curve patterns were divided into five types. A fusion level should be selected to minimise the length of fusion and yet obtain a balanced stable curve on long-term follow-up. Recommendations were made for each of the five types of curve.

3. Method of Fusion

Akbarnia BA **Selection of methodology in surgical treatment of adolescent idiopathic scoliosis** Orthop Clin North Am 1988;19:319–329

103

Dickson RA, Leatherman KD **Spinal deformities** In: Dickson RA, ed. Spinal surgery: science and practice. London: Butterworths, 1990:388–399

Mielke CH, Lonstein JE, Dennis F, Vandenbrink K, Winter RB **Surgical treatment of adolescent idiopathic scoliosis: a comparative analysis** J Bone Joint Surg [Am] 1989;71A:1170–1177

The authors appreciate that methods of instrumentation and fusion are undergoing considerable analysis and evolution at the present time. In these circumstances, references for technique will not be discussed. Three references have been chosen, largely related to principles of treatment. **Akbarnia** discussed the various methods available, assessing correction, quality of fixation and safety. The Harrington distraction rod group had a 0.23% incidence of neurological complications. Sublaminar wiring carried four times the risk, and Cotrel–Dubousset instrumentation three times the risk of the Harrington distraction group. An anterior approach using the Zielke instrumentation is ideal for a thoracolumbar curve, gives excellent correction and preserves more mobility than posterior instrumentation. **Dickson** summarised the various forms of instrumentation, discussing the Harrington instrumentation with distraction, the Zielke anterior fixation, the Luque sublaminar wiring and the Leeds procedure. The principle of the Cotrel–Dubousset instrumentation, first performed in 1983, was outlined. The need for spinal fusion and practical principles for producing a satisfactory fusion mass were discussed. **Mielke** compared the results of posterior spinal fusion in 352 patients performed between 1960 and 1984 using four types of Harrington instrumentation. No significant difference was found amongst the four groups in correction obtained at operation or final correction later.

4. The Rib Hump

Weatherley CR, Draycott V. O'Brien JF, Benson DR, Gopalakrishna KC, Evans JH, O'Brien JP **The rib deformity in adolescent idiopathic scoliosis: a prospective study to evaluate changes after Harrington distraction and posterior fusion** J Bone Joint Surg [Br] 1987;69B:179–182

Weatherley performed a prospective study in 47 patients to investigate the changes in the rib deformity after correction of the lateral curvature using Harrington distraction and posterior fusion. Despite operative correction of the lateral curve, there was a progression of the rib deformity in 64% after 4 years. Correction of the lateral curve may thus have no effect on vertebral rotation.

5. Neurological Complications

Wilber RG, Thompson GH, Shaffer JW, Brown RH, Nash CL **Postoperative neurological deficits in segmental spinal instrumentation: a study using spinal cord monitoring** J Bone Joint Surg [Am] 1984;66A:1178–1187

Wilber analysed retrospectively the postoperative neurological complications in 137 patients who underwent posterior fusion for scoliosis using different techniques. Somatosensory cortical evoked potential monitoring was employed. Three patients had a major injury to the spinal cord, and 9 patients had transient sensory changes. There was an increased risk to the spinal cord with segmental spinal instrumentation with sublaminar wires in thoracolumbar curves. Surgical correction exceeding the preoperative bending curve may also be a risk factor. Intraoperative spinal monitoring was highly accurate in predicting major spinal cord injury, but was inconsistent in predicting transient cord changes.

Spinal Cord Monitoring

Nash CL, Brown RH **Current concepts review: spinal cord monitoring** J Bone Joint Surg [Am] 1989;71A:627–630

Jones SJ, Edgar MA, Ransford AO, Thomas NP **A system for the electrophysiological monitoring of the spinal cord during operations for scoliosis** J Bone Joint Surg [Br] 1983;65B:134–139

Nash reviewed current practice in spinal cord monitoring. A standardised approach has not yet been established, but it is now routine practice to conduct some form of monitoring in performing any spinal operation associated with a high risk of neurological complications. Somatosensory cortical evoked potentials continue to be the most widely used by North American spinal surgeons, but interpretation and evaluation remains controversial. False negative and false positives are reported. The gold standard is still the wake-up test. **Jones** described the positioning of recording electrodes in the epidural space cephalad to the area to be fused. Recordings were made in response to stimulation of the posterior tibial nerve at the knee. Results in 138 patients were presented and the findings in 3 patients who exhibited neurological defects were described. It was concluded that these potentials are sensitive to minor spinal cord impairment and may be reversed when the cause is quickly remedied.

Adult Scoliosis

Bradford DS **Adult scoliosis: current concepts of treatment** Clin Orthop 1988;229:70–87

Sponseller PD, Cohen MS, Nachemson AL, Hall JE, Wohl MEB **Results of surgical treatment of adults with idiopathic scoliosis** J Bone Joint Surg [Am] 1987;69A:667–675

Bradford noted that assessment of the adult patient with scoliosis is difficult. There is controversy as to whether the incidence of back pain in the adult patient with scoliosis is greater than in an age-matched control population. Indications for treatment include curve progression, radicular pain, deterioration of pulmonary function and deformity. The benefits outweigh the risks but it must be appreciated that surgical treatment is difficult and the complication rate high. **Sponseller** discussed the outcome of surgical treatment in 45 adults who were more than 25 years old and observed for more than 3 years. The number who were free of pain was not increased after surgery. There was a 20% incidence of major complications. The limited gains to be derived from spinal fusion should be clearly explained to patients before the procedure is undertaken. It should be stressed that both these papers were produced from specialised departments with expertise in spinal surgery.

Scoliosis in Neuromuscular Disease

Cerebral Palsy

Fergusson RL, Allen BL **Considerations in the treatment of cerebral palsy patients with spinal deformities** Orthop Clin North Am 1988;19:2:419–425

Rinsky LA **Surgery of spine deformity in cerebral palsy: 12 years in the evolution of scoliosis management** Clin Orthop 1990;253:100–109

Fergusson discussed the unique problems of cerebral palsy. Progression of the deformity may occur after skeletal maturity. Significant pseudarthrosis rates may occur after fusion, especially when posterior arthrodesis is used as the sole procedure. The cerebral palsy patient is prone to regression after surgery of any kind. **Rinsky** discussed personal lessons learned from 12 years of surgery on patients with spinal deformity. Most patients were retarded non-walkers who had total body involvement, with pelvic obliquity and severe thoracolumbar curves. Three different techniques were employed. The general trend was towards longer fusion with a two-stage anterior discectomy and fusion, followed by posterior fusion. The Luque rod procedure consisting in instrumentation without fusion has been abandoned.

Duchenne Muscular Dystrophy

Shapiro F, Bresnan MJ **Current concepts review: orthopaedic management of childhood neuromuscular disease. III. Diseases of muscle** J Bone Joint Surg [Am] 1982;64A:1102–1107

Smith AD, Koreska J, Moseley CF **Progression of scoliosis in Duchenne muscular dystrophy** J Bone Joint Surg [Am] 1989;71A:1066–1074

Shapiro summarised knowledge and the orthopaedic management of patients with this disease. They rarely survive beyond late teens. The disease only involves males and demonstrates recessive inheritance. Scoliosis rarely develops while the patient is able to walk and for most an appropriate spinal orthosis is all that is necessary. The major question concerns the advisability of spinal fusion. It may be justified in a teenager for relatively longer life expectancy. **Smith** described the progression of scoliosis in 50 patients. All developed scoliosis and most of the curves were severe. When this occurred, sitting was difficult and accompanied by a breakdown of skin and pain. When walking becomes impossible, routine spinal arthrodesis should be considered.

Neurofibromatosis

Hsu LCS, Lee PC, Leong JCY **Dystrophic spinal deformities in neurofibromatosis: treatment by anterior and posterior fusion** J Bone Joint Surg [Br] 1984;66B:495–499

Calvert PT, Edgar MA, Webb PJ **Scoliosis in neurofibromatosis: the natural history with and without operation** J Bone Joint Surg [Br] 1989;71B:246–251

Crawford AH **Pitfalls of spinal deformities associated with neurofibromatosis in children** Clin Orthop 1989;245:29–42

Hsu described the results of anterior and posterior fusion for dystrophic spinal deformity in 13 patients. The morbidity rate was high in patients with angular kyphoscoliosis. Combined anterior and posterior spinal fusion may fail to control the progressive deformity. **Calvert** reviewed 47 patients with neurofibromatosis and dystrophic spinal deformities. The natural history was discussed. The most common pattern of deformity was a short angular thoracic scoliosis. Progression was usual but the rate was variable and unpredictable. Severe dystrophic changes have a poor prognosis for deterioration. **Crawford** amplified the many problems which may be encountered in the treatment of spinal deformities associated with these patients prior to surgical treatment. MRI assessment was recommended of any areas demonstrated by CT myelography to be suspect of previously unrecognised lesions. The most dangerous situation for the neurologically intact patient and the surgeon is the instrumentation and distraction of the spine in neurofibromatosis, in the presence of unrecognised intraspinal lesions.

Scheuermann's Disease

Sachs B, Bradford D, Winter R, Lonstein J, Moe J, Willson S **Scheuermann kyphosis: follow-up of Milwaukee-brace treatment** J Bone Joint Surg [Am] 1987;69A:50–57

Bradford DS, Ahmed KB, Moe JH, Winter RB, Lonstein JE **The surgical management of patients with Scheuermann's disease: a review of 24 cases managed by combined anterior and posterior fusion** J Bone Joint Surg [Am] 1980;62A:705–712

Lowe TG **Current concepts review: Scheuermann disease** J Bone Joint Surg [Am] 1990;72A:940–945

Sachs studied the long-term results of 120 patients who had used the Milwaukee brace and found it an effective method of treatment. Some loss of correction occurred with time, but the final result showed improvement in 69% followed for more than 5 years. An initial kyphosis of more than 74° required a spinal fusion. **Bradford** described the results of 24 patients who underwent correction of the deformity through a combined anterior and posterior fusion. Deformity was improved in all patients. The technique and results are illustrated. **Lowe** reviewed the aetiology, clinical and radiographic findings. Postural kyphosis is differentiated from Scheuermann disease by a less acutely angulated kyphosis and the absence of wedging of the vertebral bodies. Scheuermann disease can almost always be managed successfully with bracing if the treatment is initiated before skeletal maturity. An operation should be considered in adolescence when the deformity cannot be controlled by bracing, and in adults who have a kyphosis of 60° or more. The Cotrel–Dubousset instrumentation is being tried for operative treatment at the present time.

Tuberculosis of the Spine

Clinical Studies

Tuli SM **Results of treatment of spinal tuberculosis by "middle path regime"** J Bone Joint Surg [Br] 1975;57B:13–23

Griffiths DLl **The treatment of spinal tuberculosis** In: McKibbin B, ed. Recent advances in orthopaedics 3. Edinburgh: Churchill Livingstone, 1979: 1–17

Medical Research Council Working Party on Tuberculosis of the Spine **A 10-year assessment of a controlled trial comparing debridement and anterior spinal fusion in the management of tuberculosis of the spine in patients on standard chemotherapy in Hong Kong – Eighth report** J Bone Joint Surg [Br] 1982;64B: 393–398

Medical Research Council Working Party on Tuberculosis of the Spine **A 10-year assessment of controlled trials of inpatient and outpatient treatment and of plaster-of-Paris jackets for tuberculosis of the spine in children on standard chemotherapy. Studies in Masan and Pusan, Korea – Ninth report** J Bone Joint Surg [Br] 1985;67B:103–110

Fang D, Leong JCY, Fang HSY **Tuberculosis of the upper cervical spine** J Bone Joint Surg [Br] 1983;65B1–5:47–50

Hsu LCS, Leong JCY **Tuberculosis of the lower cervical spine (C2 to C7): a report on 40 cases** J Bone Joint Surg [Br] 1984;66B:1–5

Lifeso RM, Weaver P, Harder EH **Tuberculous spondylisis in adults** J Bone Joint Surg [Am] 1985;67A:1405–1413

Babhulkar SS, Tayade WB, Babhulkar SK **Atypical spinal tuberculosis** J Bone Joint Surg [Br] 1984;66B:239–242

Over the last 2 decades, divergent philosophies of the management of tuberculosis of the spine have been prevalent. Some have advocated surgical extirpation of every vertebral lesion whilst others claim impressive results from treatment by antitubercular drugs and rest alone. **Tuli** has tested a "middle path" regimen with antitubercular drugs and operation only for those patients, with or without neural complications, who failed to respond to drug therapy. Absolute indications for surgery were reduced to 6% without neurological complications and to 60% with neurological deficit. Ninety-four per cent of cases without neurological complication can achieve clinical healing with this regimen. The results obtained by this "middle path" regimen compare favourably with those of radical operation. In 1979, **Griffiths** debated principles of treatment, including the detailed selection of chemotherapy and the results of chemotherapy alone. Operative treatment was either limited focal surgery or radical excision, as developed in Hong Kong. The results of various controlled trials carried out under the auspices of the Medical Research Council were described. The radical operation was recommended if, and only if, surgical expertise, anaesthetic facilities and skilled nursing were available. If these were not available, reliance should be placed with confidence on ambulant outpatient therapy. Two more recent **Medical Research Council** reports have been included to provide detailed evidence on the results of differing methods of treatment. **The Eighth Report** (1982) compared radical resection of the lesion and autologous anterior bone grafts with debridement of the spinal focus without grafting. All received the same chemotherapy. Results were compared 10 years later. There was little difference between the two series and essentially all had a favourable status with a high incidence of bony fusion and no sinus formation. **The Ninth Report** (1985) compared inpatient and outpatient treatment and plaster jackets for tuberculosis of the spine in children on standard chemotherapy. The results confirmed the effectiveness of PAS plus isoniazid in achieving quiescence in spinal tuberculosis, even in patients ambulatory from the start of chemotherapy. The study demonstrated no benefit from immobilisation, either by initial bed rest or a plaster-of-Paris jacket. **Fang** described 6 patients, aged between 3 and 51 years, with tuberculosis of the upper cervical spine. Prominent features included pain and stiffness, paralysis, swelling of the retropharyngeal soft tissue, osteolytic erosions and atlantoaxial subluxation. Cure was obtained with antibiotics, transoral depression and C1–2 fusion. **Hsu** reviewed 40 patients with tuberculosis of the lower cervical spine. Pain and stiffness were important dominant symptoms. Two types of disease were noted. In children under 10, involvement was extensive, with large abscesses. In children over 10, the disease was localised but with a higher incidence of Pott's paraplegia. Cord compression occurred in 40%. Treatment was with antituberculous drugs, anterior excision and bone grafts. This relieved pain, Pott's paraplegia, and corrected the kyphosis. **Lifeso** described experience in the treatment of 107 adults with spinal tuberculosis in Saudi Arabia. Diagnosis was often difficult, with negative bone and gallium scans. Neurological recovery and relief of pain occurred more rapidly in the surgically treated group. There were no organisms that were resistant to isoniazid, rifampicin or ethambutol. Neither progression nor reactivation of disease occurred after 12 months of adequate chemotherapy. **Babhulkar** drew attention to patients with spinal tuberculosis in India, who present without characteristic destruction of adjacent vertebral bodies and with no deformity, and yet with symptoms and signs of cord compression. There were two groups: those with tuberculosis of the neural arch and those with extraosseous extradural tuberculosis. Both may require laminectomy.

Pott's Paraplegia

Hodgson AR, Skinsnes OK, Leong CY **The pathogenesis of Pott's paraplegia** J Bone Joint Surg [Am] 1967;49A:1147–1156

Hsu LCS, Cheng CL, Leong CY **Pott's Paraplegia of late onset. The cause of compression and results after anterior decompression** J Bone Joint Surg [Br] 1988;70B:534–538

Hodgson in 1967 reviewed the pathogenesis of Pott's paraplegia. While acknowledging the well-known causes, such as abscess or granulation tissue in active disease and bone pressure in healed disease, Hodgson stressed the intrinsic causes due to tuberculous infection passing through the barrier of the coverings of the spinal cord. This may produce irreversible paraplegia. There is an urgent need to perform adequate decompression in Pott's paraplegia. **Griffiths** (see above) considered that the time-honoured distinction between paraplegia of early onset and paraplegia of late onset is less important than it was. Although many cases of paraplegia in active disease will respond to conservative treatment, nevertheless there are strong arguments for operative decompression of all cases showing severe involvement of the central nervous system in active spinal tuberculosis. The technique must include full exposure of the front of the dura at the apex of the kyphus. Griffiths advocated that the best method of decompression is the Hong Kong radical anterior resection. **Hsu** analysed the cause of compression in 22 patients with late onset paraplegia, presenting a mean of 18 years after initial symptoms. Fourteen had active disease, usually at the apex of the kyphus. In the remainder with healed disease, hard bony ridges compressed the spinal cord. The response to surgery was faster and better with active disease.

Secondary Tumours of the Spine

Kostuik JP, Errico TJ, Gleason TF, Errico CC **Spine stabilization of vertebral column tumors** Spine 1988;13:250–256

Turner PL, Prince HG, Webb JK, Sokal MPJW **Surgery for malignant extradural tumours of the spine** J Bone Joint Surg [Br] 1988;70B:451–456

Galasko CSB **Spinal instability secondary to metastatic cancer** J Bone Joint Surg [Br] 1991;73B:104–108

Kostuik analysed indications, techniques and results of stabilization and decompression of 100 consecutive spinal tumours. Localised metastatic disease is best approached anteriorly. A primary tumour is best treated by en bloc resection. The unstable spine often requires stabilization for pain relief. The merits of anterior and posterior approaches were debated. In malignant disease, cement provided stability in 87 of 91 procedures. **Turner** reviewed 41 patients with malignant extradural tumours treated by anterior decompression for cord compression, uncontrolled back pain or both. An anterior operation achieved major neurological recovery in 56% with neurological loss. No patient with complete paraplegia gained a useful recovery. Back pain was usually improved. **Galasko** discussed experience with 55 patients with severe pain caused by spinal instability. Alleviation of pain and restoration of mobility were best achieved by segmental spinal stabilization using the Hartshill rectangle or the Banks–Dervin rod. A few patients required a combined anterior and posterior stabilization. Postoperative radiotherapy is recommended with appropriate endocrine or chemotherapy. Posterior stabilization is at least as effective in the control of spinal instability as an anterior approach.

Section 5
The Lower Limb

Limb-Length Inequality

The Classic

Green WT, Anderson M **Epiphyseal arrest for the correction of discrepancies in length of the lower extremities** J Bone Joint Surg [Am] 1957;39A:853–872

In 1957, **Green** summarised experience of 475 operations to correct discrepancy in the length of the lower extremities by inhibition of growth; of these, 383 were by epiphysiodesis and 92 by stapling. The majority were observed for many years until growth was completed. The timing of arrest was based on the classic prediction charts previously published by the two authors in 1947. Epiphysiodesis and stapling were both shown to be effective procedures for correcting limb-length discrepancy providing they were used correctly. Complications were discussed but generally these were minor. The merits and disadvantages of the two procedures were debated in detail.

Basic Studies

Moseley CF **A straight-line graph for leg-length discrepancies** J Bone Joint Surg [Am] 1977;59A:174–179

Shapiro F **Developmental patterns in lower-extremity length discrepancies** J Bone Joint Surg [Am] 1982;64A:639–651

Moseley in 1977 described a graphic method which facilitates and provides interpretation of data in cases of leg-length discrepancy. It provided a mechanism for predicting future growth which automatically took into account the child's growth percentile and the degree of inhibition in the short leg. The method is more accurate than the prediction charts of Green and Anderson. Growth of the short leg was represented by a straight line which lay below that of the long leg and may have a different slope. **Shapiro** in 1982 reviewed lower-extremity length discrepancy data in 802 patients, and demonstrated that not all discrepancies continue to increase at a constant rate with time. Developmental discrepancy patterns were identified and presented. Determination of the distribution of pattern types in various conditions aids growth prediction, and in conjunction with the Green and Anderson charts, permits accurate projections of discrepancy.

Clinical Studies

Hood RW, Riseborough EJ **Lengthening of the lower extremity by the Wagner method. A review of the Boston Children's Hospital experience** J Bone Joint Surg [Am] 1981;63A:1122–1131

Winquist RA, Hansen ST, Pearson RE **Closed intramedullary shortening of the femur** Clin Orthop 1978;136:54–61

Wilde GP, Baker GCW **Circumferential periosteal release in the treatment of children with leg-length inequality** J Bone Joint Surg [Br] 1987;69B:817–821

De Bastiani G, Aldegheri R, Brivio LR, Trivella G **Chondrodiatasis-controlled symmetrical distraction of the epiphyseal plate. Limb lengthening in children** J Bone Joint Surg [Br] 1986;68B:550–556

Aldegheri R, Brivio LR, Agostini S **The callotasis method of limb lengthening** Clin Orthop 1989;241:137–145

Aldegheri R, Trivella G, Renzi-Brivio L, Tessari G, Agostini S, Lavini F **Lengthening of the lower limbs in achondroplastic patients: a comparative study of four techniques** J Bone Joint Surg [Br] 1988;70B:69–73

The management of appreciable leg-length inequality is still controversial. Studies are presented which summarise problems and trends. **Hood** described the results of experience with 40 lengthenings of the leg, both femoral and tibial. The overall complication rate was high (92%) but it did not significantly affect the ultimate goal of equalisation of limb length. The authors considered the Wagner method to be the procedure of choice for continuous distraction lengthening when the severity of limb-length discrepancy merits major surgical intervention. Based on experience with 40 patients, **Windquist** concluded that closed intramedullary shortening of the femur in the adult provided a method of equalisation that posed minimal operative risks and provided an excellent functional and cosmetic result. Shortening averaged 3.3 cm. Three patients had significant complications. The technique is demanding. The results of 38 children with leg inequality treated by circumferential periosteal release were presented by **Wilde**. The children were considered to be too young for structural lengthening but had a predicted discrepancy of over 3 cm. All patients showed a decrease in the percentage difference between the two limbs at 1 year after operation, the size of the response being more pronounced in younger children. The method was considered reliable and safe and a useful addition to the methods of treatment of limb inequality.

   De Bastiani described a technique for slow progressive symmetrical distraction of the growth plate using an axial fixation system. The aim was to preserve growth plate function and gain length. Experiences were described with both leg-length discrepancy and achondroplasia. The method was considered to be the least traumatic available for lengthening. Complications were minimal and the child was able to walk and attend school while the fixation was in place. Callotasis is a lengthening technique that involves slow, controlled distraction after sub-periosteal sub-metaphyseal osteotomy. **Aldegheri** (1989) described the technique and its advantages over other methods; the results of 270 bone segment operations were discussed. **Aldegheri** (1988) reported remarkable experience of lengthening by over 30% a total of 117 lower limbs in achondroplastic patients. Chondrodiatasis of the femur and callotasis of the tibia were the techniques which gave fewest complications.

The Ilizarov Technique

Ilizarov GA **Clinical application of the tension–stress effect for limb lengthening** Clin Orthop 1990;250:8–26

Paley D **Problems, obstacles and complications of limb lengthening by the Ilizarov technique** Clin Orthop 1990;250:81–104

Ilizarov described the development of a system of orthopaedics, traumatology and limb lengthening using a circular transfixation wire external skeletal fixator, associated with a biomechanical method of stimulating new osseous tissue within a widening osteotomy distraction site. Stable fixation of bone fragments is the most important principle in clinical application, yet it permits full weight bearing and physiological function of the entire limb. The wide clinical application is discussed including lengthening of 400 achondroplastic dwarfs. In a symposium on limb lengthening, **Paley** narrated experience with this technique with 46 patients. Although this technique is a more physiological method of lengthening than the Wagner, there were still many problems. There were 10 major complications, but the original goals of surgery were achieved in 57 of the 60 segments treated.

Review Article

Siffert RS **Current concepts review: lower limb-length discrepancy** J Bone Joint Surg [Am] 1987;69A:1100–1106

Siffert comprehensively reviewed analysis and treatment of limb-length discrepancy. He stressed that limb-lengthening procedures are demanding of clinical judgement and technical skill, and are not procedures for the occasional surgeon. All of the methods of femoral shortening appear to be equally effective but are associated with the same potential complications. To maintain the integrity of the ankle joint, screw fixation at the distal part of the fibula is necessary before tibial lengthening is undertaken. The final decision as to the most desirable treatment demands careful debate of the alternatives between patient, relatives and surgeon.

Ogden JA Current concepts review: the evaluation and treatment of partial physeal arrest J Bone Joint Surg [Am] 1987;69A:1297–1302

Closure of the growth plate may lead to problems of limb inequality. This subject was previously considered under the title "The Growth Plate" in *Selected References in Orthopaedic Trauma* ed Ratliff AHC, Dixon JH, Magnussen PA, Young SK (page 24). **Ogden** provides a rapid reference and therefore this paper is included at the end of this section.

Tarsal Tunnel Syndrome

Kaplan PE, Kernahan WT **Tarsal tunnel syndrome: an electrodiagnostic and surgical correlation** J Bone Joint Surg [Am] 1981;63A:96–99

Kaplan discussed the diagnosis and treatment of the tarsal tunnel syndrome, based on a study of 21 patients. All had burning pain and paraesthesiae with tenderness posterior to the medial malleolus over the posterior tibial nerve. Electrodiagnostic evaluation showed that reduced amplitude and increased duration of motor evoked potentials was a more sensitive indicator of this condition than distal motor latency. Surgical release resulted in complete relief.

The Hip

Congenital Dislocation

Early Diagnosis, Screening and Treatment

Barlow TG **Early diagnosis and treatment of congenital dislocation of the hip** J Bone Joint Surg [Br] 1962;44B:292–301

Dunn PM, Evans RE, Thearle MJ, Griffiths HED, Witherow PJ **Congenital dislocation of the hip: early and late diagnosis and management compared** Arch Dis Child 1985;60:407–414

Berman L, Klenerman L **Ultrasound screening for hip abnormalities: preliminary findings in 1001 neonates** Br Med J 1986;293:719–722

Clarke NMP, Clegg J, Al-Chalabi AN **Ultrasound screening of hips at risk for CDH: failure to reduce the incidence of late cases** J Bone Joint Surg [Br] 1989;71B:9–12

Jones DA, Powell N **Ultrasound and neonatal hip screening: a prospective study of high risk babies** J Bone Joint Surg [Br] 1990;72B:457-459

Ozonoff MB **The radiological assessment of congenital dislocation of the hip** Curr Orthop 1987;1:258–266

Ferguson AB (Jr) **Congenital dislocation of the hip: treatment in infants.** In: Galasko CSB, Noble J, eds. Current trends in orthopaedic surgery. Manchester: Manchester University Press, 1988:176–197

In 1962 **Barlow** described a test more sensitive than Ortolani's for the diagnosis of instability of the hip in the newborn. About one infant in 60 is born with instability of one or both hips. A small percentage (12%) are true congenital dislocations and persist unless treated. **Dunn** reported the results of clinical studies on 23 002 infants screened for the possibility of congenital dislocation of the hip. Where a hip abnormality was detected, immediate treatment in an abduction splint was undertaken. Only 1% required further orthopaedic treatment. These results were compared with those of 91 cases of late congenital dislocation of the hip, 7 of whom required open surgery. Controversy continues concerning the place of neonatal screening in the detection of CDH. There is little doubt that ultrasound examination is an accurate method of diagnosing CDH in infancy. Three papers have been included which debate these problems. **Berman** discussed the value of routine screening. Clinically normal but dysplastic hips exist and ultrasound will detect them. Such detection may prevent overtreatment. The paper contains clear illustrations of the four types of appearance classified by Graf. **Clarke** described the results of assessment of 4617 babies born in Coventry in 1986 and examined by ultrasound. Three late cases of CDH presented among the babies born in 1986, but these had not been examined by ultrasound. Ultrasound screening in 1986 had therefore failed to reduce the incidence of late cases. **Jones** used ultrasound screening for 812 hips in babies with a "high risk factor". It is suggested that a large proportion of the potential late cases are contained within the extended high risk group, but clearly it is still necessary to study at birth, by ultrasound, a complete population in order to define more accurately the precise importance of this high risk group. **Ozonoff** debated various methods and values of radiological assessment, including standard radiography, ultrasonography and arthrography. Computed tomography is useful to assess therapeutic results and plan later operative treatment. The place of magnetic resonance imaging is still unclear. **Ferguson** has provided a recent review of the various problems that cause concern in the treatment of infants; he particularly discussed the value and results of treatment where an open reduction had been employed through the medial approach. Seventy-seven cases were studied with a minimum follow-up of 10 years.

Aetiology

Wynne Davies R **Acetabular dysplasia and familial joint laxity: two aetiological factors in congenital dislocation of the hip. A review of 589 patients and their families** J Bone Joint Surg [Br] 1970;52B:704–716

Wynne Davies surveyed the genetic and other aetiological factors in 589 patients with congenital dislocation of the hip and their families. Two aetiological groups were described, one with acetabular dysplasia inherited as a multiple gene system and another with joint laxity responsible for a high proportion of neonatal cases.

Treatment – Young Child

MacKenzie IG, Seddon HJ, Trevor D **Congenital dislocation of the hip** J Bone Joint Surg [Br] 1960;42B:689–705

Somerville EW, Scott JC **The direct approach to congenital dislocation of the hip** J Bone Joint Surg [Br] 1957;39B:623–640

Gibson PH, Benson MKD **Congenital dislocation of the hip: review at maturity of 147 hips treated by excision of the limbus and derotation osteotomy** J Bone Joint Surg [Br] 1982;64B:169–175

Lindstrom JR, Ponseti IV, Wenger DR **Acetabular development after reduction in congenital dislocation of the hip** J Bone Joint Surg [Am] 1979; 61A: 112–118

Kasser JR, Bowen JR, MacEwen GD **Varus derotation osteotomy in the treatment of persistent dysplasia in congenital dislocation of the hip** J Bone Joint Surg [Am] 1985;67A:195–202

Salter RB, Dubos J-P **The first 15 years' personal experience with innominate osteotomy in the treatment of congenital dislocation and subluxation of the hip** Clin Orthop 1974; 98:72–103

In 1960, **MacKenzie** reviewed the results of treatment of 167 hips at the Royal National Orthopaedic Hospital, London, followed for at least 5 years. Closed reduction gave "reasonably satisfactory and durable results in a fair proportion of cases"; it could succeed up to the age of 5 years. The pathology and anatomical barriers to closed reduction were discussed. In 1957, **Somerville** developed his method of treatment of the congenitally dislocated hip, believing that structural abnormalities should be corrected by early open reduction followed by medial rotation osteotomy. The importance of arthrography, detection of the limbus and its removal were stressed. **Gibson** recently reviewed at maturity 147 cases treated by this regimen. Attention was focused on the good and bad prognostic factors. The most serious problem was the premature onset of degenerative arthritis even in hips which seemed to have been satisfactorily reduced. **Lindstrom** studied acetabular development in 185 congenitally dislocated hips. Early treatment led to the best acetabular development which continued up to the age of 8 years providing the femoral head remained concentrically reduced. The indications and limitations of varus derotation osteotomy for persistent dysplasia were studied in 34 patients (44 hips) by **Kasser**. Consistently good results occurred in patients less than 4 years old at the time of operation. Results were less predictable as the patients approached the age of 8. **Salter** has reviewed his outstanding experience with pelvic osteotomy, discussing in detail the indications, contraindications, technique and results.

Avascular Necrosis

Kalamchi A, MacEwen GD **Avascular necrosis following treatment of congenital dislocation of the hip** J Bone Joint Surg [Am] 1980;62A:876–888

Four patterns of vascular changes involving the femoral head and capital epiphyseal plate were described by **Kalamchi**. The end results in skeletally mature patients following avascular necrosis in childhood were discussed. The more severe forms of necrosis were found in those patients where treatment was begun between birth and the age of 6 months. Preliminary traction reduced the incidence of the more severe cases of necrosis.

Treatment – Older Child

Summers BN, Turner A, Wynn-Jones CH **The shelf operation in the management of late presentation of congenital hip dysplasia** J Bone Joint Surg [Br] 1988;70B:63–68

Pozo JL, Cannon SR, Catterall A **The Colonna–Hey–Groves arthroplasty in the late treatment of congenital dislocation of the hip – a long-term review** J Bone Joint Surg [Br] 1987;69B:220–228

Hogh J, Macnicol MF **The Chiari pelvic osteotomy: a long-term review of clinical and radiographic results** J Bone Joint Surg [Br] 1987;69B:365–373

Reynolds DA **Chiari innominate osteotomy in adults – technique, indications and contraindications** J Bone Joint Surg [Br] 1986;68B:45–54

Review Article

Coleman SS **Reconstructive procedures in congenital dislocation of the hip**
In: McKibbin B, ed. Recent advances in orthopaedics 4. Edinburgh: Churchill
Livingstone, 1983:23–43

Many surgical procedures have been described for the treatment of congenital hip
dysplasia after early childhood. We have chosen five articles in an endeavour to
summarise this difficult problem. **Summers** described the results of the shelf
operation performed on 24 patients with a mean follow-up of 16 years. The operation
is safe; good cover is provided for the femoral head and adequate support for the
possible seating of an acetabular prosthesis. Forty-four patients who had undergone
50 capsular arthroplasties were reviewed by **Pozo** after a mean follow-up of 20 years.
The operation aims to relocate the capsule-covered femoral head within a surgically
deepened acetabulum. Seventy per cent of the hips showed good function despite a
reduced range of movement. **Hogh** reviewed 94 Chiari medial displacement
osteotomies after a mean follow-up of 10 years. Where the indication for surgery
was pain, over 80% had appreciable relief in the short term. The osteotomy
effectively stabilises the fulcrum of the hip joint. Various useful details of technique
were noted. **Reynolds** reported experience and results of 44 Chiari osteotomies in
39 adult patients, the average age being 35 years. Four categories of dysplasia and
degeneration were described and careful preoperative selection stressed. The
operation is stated to be safe, not difficult and less demanding than the complex
alternative "double" and "triple" osteotomies. **Coleman**, in a review article,
discussed the various reconstructive procedures that may be employed for congenital
dislocation of the hip. The advantages and disadvantages of various pelvic
osteotomies were discussed, including the Pemberton, Salter, Sutherland and "Dial".
The considerable controversy concerning the indications for and value of varus
and rotational osteotomies of the femur was also outlined.

Perthes' Disease

Classification

Catterall A **The natural history of Perthes' disease** J Bone Joint Surg [Br]
1971;53B:37–53

Christensen F, Soballe K, Ejsted R, Luxhoj T **The Catterall classification of
Perthes' disease: an assessment of reliability** J Bone Joint Surg [Br] 1986;68B:
614–615

In 1971, **Catterall** classified the severity of involvement of the epiphysis into four groups and noted that the prognosis was related to that severity. The concept of a "head at risk" was introduced. Those patients with mild disease (groups I and II), especially in the younger age groups, will obtain a good result without treatment, and this applies to some 50% of patients. **Christensen** checked the reliability of the Catterall grouping in 100 hip joints whose radiographs were studied by four experienced observers. There was a significant and unacceptable disagreement in assessment, and he questioned whether the Catterall classification should form the basis for decisions of treatment .

Aetiology and Pathogenesis

Landin LA, Danielsson LG, Wattsgard C **Transient synovitis of the hip: its incidence, epidemiology and relation to Perthes' disease** J Bone Joint Surg [Br] 1987;69B:238–242

Inoue A, Freeman MAR, Vernon-Roberts B, Mizuno S **The pathogenesis of Perthes' disease** J Bone Joint Surg [Br] 1976;58B:453–461

Harrison MHM, Turner MH, Jacobs P **Skeletal immaturity in Perthes' disease** J Bone Joint Surg [Br] 1976;58B:37–40

Hall AJ, Barker DJP **Perthes' disease in Yorkshire** J Bone Joint Surg [Br] 1989;71B:229–233

The possible relation of Perthes' disease to traumatic synovitis of the hip has been analysed by **Landin**, based on a prospective study of 294 episodes of acute transient synovitis of the hip. Perthes' disease followed the acute synovitis in only 3.4%. In 1976, **Inoue** described the histological appearance of 57 femoral head biopsy specimens in Perthes' disease. In one-half, appearances characteristic of double infarction were present. This concept might explain the deformation and chronicity of this condition. In the same journal, **Harrison** drew attention to the constitutional nature of Perthes' disease. The skeletal age of 182 children suffering from this disease was analysed, and delayed skeletal maturation was noted. The evidence for geographical variations in the incidence of this condition was debated by **Hall** who found that these variations could not be explained by urban–rural or social class differences.

Long-term Follow-up

Ratliff AHC **Perthes' disease. II. The long-term results** In: Lloyd-Roberts GC, Ratliff AHC. Hip disorders in children. London: Butterworths, 1978:150–164

Brotherton BJ, McKibbin B **Perthes' disease treated by prolonged recumbency and femoral head containment: a long-term appraisal** J Bone Joint Surg [Br] 1977;59B:8–14

McAndrew MP, Weinstein SL **A long-term follow-up of Legg-Calve-Perthes' disease** J Bone Joint Surg [Am] 1984;66A:860–869

Ratliff reported a long-term study of patients observed into adult life. Even those healing with deformed femoral heads fared surprisingly well 3 or 4 decades later. **Brotherton** described a long-term review of 102 hips treated by a rigorous conservative regimen with the hips contained by "broomstick" plasters; 88% of results were classified as good. Benefit was important especially in those where the femoral head was totally involved (group IV). **McAndrew** traced 112 patients observed for an average of almost 50 years. If a spherical head is obtained by adult life, a good functional result may be expected. A deformed femoral head may lead to satisfactory function for many years, but 50% of patients in this study had disabling osteoarthrosis by the time they reached the 6th decade of life.

The Difficult Hip

Clarke NMP, Harrison MHM **Painful sequelae of coxa plana** J Bone Joint Surg [Am] 1983;65A:13–18

Quain S, Catterall A **Hinge abduction of the hip: diagnosis and treatment** J Bone Joint Surg [Br] 1986;68B:61–64

Clarke discussed the problems presented by 31 patients with an average age of 27 years, who had painful hips as a result of coxa plana in childhood. The series was presented to show that Perthes' disease may be followed by major disability within the first 3 decades of life. Cases were collected in a special clinic in Birmingham. **Quain** has developed the concept of hinge abduction of the hip, i.e. the abnormal movement which may develop when a deformed femoral head impinges on the lateral lip of the acetabulum. The diagnosis and treatment is described in 27 patients; satisfactory results were obtained using abduction extension osteotomy of the femur.

Growth Changes

Barnes JM **Premature epiphyseal closure in Perthes' disease** J Bone Joint Surg [Br] 1980;62B:432–437

Kerat D, Harrison MHM, Clarke NMP, Hall DJ **Coxa plana – the fate of the physis** J Bone Joint Surg [Am] 1984;66A:870–877

During the last few years, an increasing awareness has developed of the importance of premature fusion at the growth plate in Perthes' disease. **Barnes** stated that it was an infrequent complication, but he collected a series of 22 patients with this problem. **Kerat** considered that interference with the growth at the epiphyseal plate in Perthes' disease is more common than previously suspected. It may be revealed by over-growth of the greater trochanter, lateral protrusion of the nucleus and medial bowing of the femoral neck.

Treatment

Lloyd-Roberts GC **Editorial: the management of Perthes' disease** J Bone Joint Surg [Br] 1982;64B:1–2

Coates CJ, Paterson JMH, Woods KR, Catterall A, Fixsen JA **Femoral osteotomy in Perthes' disease: results at maturity** J Bone Joint Surg [Br] 1990; 72B:581–585

Salter RB **Current concepts review: the present status of surgical treatment for Legg–Perthes' disease** J Bone Joint Surg [Am] 1984;66A:961–966

The treatment of Perthes' disease is still controversial. **Lloyd-Roberts** has summarised the debate. There would appear to be general agreement that containment is essential, either by conservative or operative means. Treatment by abduction splints and its results has already been described by **Brotherton**. **Coates** described the results of femoral osteotomy in 44 patients at skeletal maturity. The indication for operation was Catterall Group II, III and IV hips with "head-at-risk" signs. Each hip was assigned radiographically to one of the five Stulberg classes. Results showed excellent clinical function but a positive Trendelenburg sign was seen in 25%. The results of femoral osteotomy were considered to be better than those of conservative treatment in all age groups, except those under 5 years. **Salter** has classified the various accepted forms of management and debated the arguments, including the value of pelvic osteotomy.

Slipped Upper Femoral Epiphysis

Incidence and Aetiology

Rennie AM **The inheritance of slipped upper femoral epiphysis** J Bone Joint Surg [Br] 1982;64B:180–184

Hagglund G, Hannson LI, Ordeberg G **Epidemiology of slipped capital femoral epiphysis in southern Sweden** Clin Orthop 1984;191:82–94

Gelberman RH, Cohen MS, Shaw BA, Kasser JR, Griffin PP, Wilkinson RH **The association of femoral retroversion with slipped capital femoral epiphysis** J Bone Joint Surg [Am] 1986;68A:1000–1007

Rennie has reviewed 214 cases. He suggests that the condition may be inherited as an autosomal dominant with variable penetrance. The epidemiology and incidence in southern Sweden have been studied by **Hagglund**, based on 532 cases treated at three orthopaedic departments over many years. **Gelberman** measured the degree of femoral anteversion in 25 patients who had a unilateral or bilateral slip, using computerised axial tomography. A decreased angle of femoral anteversion appeared to be associated with the development of slipped epiphysis. It is suggested that altered mechanical forces may contribute to the cause of this condition.

Classification and Remodelling

Dunn DM, Angel JC **Replacement of the femoral head by open operation in severe adolescent slipping of the upper femoral epiphysis** J Bone Joint Surg [Br] 1978;60B:394–403

O'Brien ET, Fahey JJ **Remodelling of the femoral neck after in situ pinning for slipped capital epiphysis** J Bone Joint Surg [Am] 1977;59A:62–68

Dunn classified these injuries into four types, stressing their differing prognosis. The severe acute traumatic slip, whose treatment is controversial, is very rare. Remodelling of the femoral neck with growth after pinning has been emphasised by **O'Brien**, even in patients treated for a moderate or severe slip.

Long-term Follow-up

Boyer DW, Mickelson MR, Ponseti IV **Slipped capital femoral epiphysis: long-term follow-up study of 121 patients** J Bone Joint Surg [Am] 1981;63A:85–95

The classic paper by **Boyer** and his colleagues evaluated 121 patients for a minimum of 21 years. The results were very good in most of the 83 hips with the slip left unreduced. The long-term results, even in moderate and severe slips, were better after in situ fixation than after operative or manipulative treatment.

Treatment – The Mild Slip

Stambough JL, Davidson RS, Ellis RD, Gregg JR **Slipped capital femoral epiphysis: an analysis of 80 patients as to pin placement and number** J Pediatr Orthop 1986;6:265–273

Greenough CG, Bromage JD, Jackson AM **Pinning of the slipped upper femoral epiphysis – a trouble-free procedure?** J Pediatr Orthop 1985;5: 657–660

It is widely accepted that for a slip of less than 30° pinning in situ or epiphyseodesis will give excellent results in the majority of cases. The papers by both **Stambough** and **Greenough** reflect a trend towards awareness of the need for care and skill in the accurate insertion of pins. The severity of complications increases with the number of pins used; two are probably sufficient and they must not enter the joint. Greenough noted a complication rate of 34% for the operation.

Treatment – The Severe Slip

Broughton NS, Todd RC, Dunn DM, Angel JC **Open reduction of the severely slipped upper femoral epiphysis** J Bone Joint Surg [Br] 1988;70B:435–439

Melby A, Hoyt WA, Weiner DS **Treatment of chronic slipped capital femoral epiphysis by bone-graft epiphyseodesis** J Bone Joint Surg [Am] 1980;62A: 119–125

Szypryt EP, Clement DA, Colton CL **Open reduction or epiphysiodesis for slipped upper femoral epiphysis: a comparison of Dunn's operation and the Heyman–Herndon procedure** J Bone Joint Surg [Br] 1987;69B:737–742

Rao JP, Francis AM, Siwek CW **The treatment of chronic slipped capital femoral epiphysis by biplane osteotomy** J Bone Joint Surg [Am] 1984;66A: 1169–1175

The successful treatment of moderate and severe slips remains a subject of debate. Dunn (1978) (see Classification and Remodelling) described the technique of his operation for open replacement of the femoral head and concluded that this is an excellent method of treatment for a severe chronic slip, providing the epiphyseal plate is still open. There was a greater incidence of avascular necrosis in acute-on-chronic cases; he did not advise manipu-lative reduction.

More recently, **Broughton** has reported the results of 115 of these same patients with a longer follow-up. There was a low incidence of complications, including avascular necrosis and chondrolysis. There were more complications with an acute-on-chronic slip. **Melby** described the results of 106 hips treated by bone-graft epiphyseodesis. Rapid and reliable growth plate closure occurred and there was no evidence of cartilage or bone necrosis. **Szypryt** compared the results of the Dunn operation and epiphyseodesis with surgical osteoplasty as advocated by Heyman. Dunn's open reduction gave better results for a hip with a severe slip but the Heyman-Herndon procedure was successful for moderate slips.

Many techniques of intertrochanteric and subtrochanteric osteotomy have been described for the correction of late deformity after the epiphysis has fused. We have selected the paper by **Rao**, who noted that a biplane osteotomy is not an easy procedure, but it is nevertheless forgiving. No patients had avascular necrosis of the femoral head or symptoms of degenerative arthritis at follow-up.

The Contralateral Hip

Hagglund G, Hansson LI, Ordeberg G, Sandstrom S **Bilaterality in slipped upper femoral epiphysis** J Bone Joint Surg [Br] 1988;70B:179–181

Emery RJH, Todd RC, Dunn DM **Prophylactic pinning of slipped upper femoral epiphysis: prevention of complications** J Bone Joint Surg [Br] 1990; 72B:217–219

Hagglund studied the frequency of slipping and osteoarthritis of the contralateral hip in 260 patients with slipped epiphysis between 1910 and 1960. There was a total of 61% with bilateral slips. Management of the contralateral hip is still controversial, but Hagglund concluded that, with a slipped epiphysis, prophylactic contralateral pinning should be performed to avoid slipping and reduce the risk of late osteoarthritis. **Emery** reported the complications of prophylactic pinning with Crawford–Adams pins in 95 cases. The most common complication was penetration, which occurred in 14%. There were no cases of chondrolysis or avascular necrosis. The major difficulty of pin removal was buried pins requiring excavation. Many of the complications reported could have been avoided by better surgical technique.

Complications

Ingram AJ, Clarke MS, Clark CS, Marshall WR **Chondrolysis complicating slipped capital femoral epiphysis** Clin Orthop 1982;165:99–109

Ingram has provided a comprehensive review of the perplexing complication of chondrolysis. Although apparently rare in this country, in the series from the Campbell Clinic there was an incidence of 29%.

Transient Synovitis

Kallio P, Ryoppy S, Kunnamo I **Transient synovitis and Perthes' disease: is there an aetiological connection?** J Bone Joint Surg [Br] 1986;68B:808–811

Landin LA, Danielsson LG, Wattsgard C **Transient synovitis of the hip: its incidence, epidemiology and relation to Perthes' disease** J Bone Joint Surg [Br] 1987;69B:238–242

Kallio carried out a prospective study of 119 children with transient synovitis. Perthes' disease did not develop in follow-up. However, there was moderate overgrowth of the femoral head in 33%. It was concluded that Perthes' disease does not result after elevated intra-articular pressure found in transient synovitis. **Landin** performed a prospective 5-year study of 294 episodes of acute transient synovitis of the hip. The risk of recurrence was 20 times greater than the risk of a single episode. Perthes' disease was later diagnosed in 10 cases (3%) but review of the initial radiographs showed that only two cases had had completely normal appearances.

Osteoarthritis

Pathology

(See General Section – Osteoarthritis)

Mechanics

Bombelli R, Santore RF, Poss R **Mechanics of the normal and osteoarthritic hip: a new perspective** Clin Orthop 1984;182:69–78

Bombelli considered that the essential anatomical requisite for the maintenance of mechanical equilibrium about the hip is a horizontal acetabular weight-bearing surface. Anatomical deviations from this result in a disequilibrium of opposing forces and may contribute to the onset of osteoarthritis.

Treatment – Upper Femoral Osteotomy

Nissen KI **Editorial: the arrest of primary osteoarthritis of the hip** J Bone Joint Surg [Br] 1960;42B:423–424

Harris NH, Kirwan E **The results of osteotomy for early primary osteo-arthritis of the hip** J Bone Joint Surg [Br] 1964;46B:477–487

Weisl H **Intertrochanteric osteotomy for osteoarthritis: a long-term follow-up** J Bone Joint Surg [Br] 1980;62B:37–42

Poss R **Current concepts review: the role of osteotomy in the treatment of osteoarthritis of the hip** J Bone Joint Surg [Am] 1984;66A:144–151

Bombelli R, Andrew TA, Flanagan JP **Intertrochanteric osteotomy of the hip** In: Chapman MW, ed. Operative orthopaedics, Vol 1. Philadelphia: JB Lippincott, 649–662

Book Reference

Schatzker J, ed. **The intertrochanteric osteotomy.** Berlin: Springer-Verlag, 1984

For several decades before the advent of total hip arthroplasty, upper femoral osteotomy was widely employed as the favourite method of surgical treatment of osteoarthritis of the hip. **Nissen** in 1960 championed this treatment, and indeed suggested that osteotomy might arrest progression of this condition. **Harris** described clinical and radiological results of 71 osteotomies for primary osteoarthritis of the hip performed with internal fixation and followed for 2–8 years. The review supported Nissen's suggestion that hip osteotomy should be performed early while the joint is still mobile. The possible causes of failure were discussed. **Weisl** described the results of 757 intertrochanteric osteotomies for osteoarthritis of the hip. In two-thirds of the hips the joint space was increased, and a similar proportion experienced relief of pain lasting at least 5 years. However, the effects of the osteotomy declined after 10 years and only a quarter of the hips had a lasting "good result". The best results were obtained in active patients under 70 years of age with unilateral hip disease. **Poss** reviewed the role of osteotomy with discussion of the evolution of this operation, the selection of suitable patients and the surgical technique. The arguments of osteotomy versus total hip arthroplasty were debated. The two operations should be regarded as complementary rather than competitive procedures. **Bombelli** described three types of osteoarthritis (superolateral, medial and concentric) and the indications and objectives of osteotomy. The technique of the various types of valgus and varus osteotomy were discussed. The book by **Schatzker** is commended for more detailed information on osteotomy. Attention is drawn to "Intertrochanteric Osteotomy": Muller ME, pages 25–67; "Biomechanical Classification of Osteoarthritis of the Hip": Bombelli R, Aronson J, pages 67–134.

Total Hip Arthroplasty

Historical

Eftekhar NA **An historical note on the development of hip arthroplasty** In: Principles of total hip arthroplasty. St. Louis: CV Mosby Co, 1978:1–8

Charnley J **Arthroplasty of the hip – a new operation** Lancet 1961;1:1129–1132

Charnley J **The long-term results of low-friction arthroplasty of the hip performed as a primary intervention** J Bone Joint Surg [Br] 1972;54B:61–76

Ring PA **Complete replacement arthroplasty of the hip by the Ring prosthesis** J Bone Joint Surg [Br] 1968;50B:720–731

Eftekhar provided a concise summary of the development of hip arthroplasty, including interpositional, reconstructive and replacement. The introduction of acrylic cement and high-density polythene as materials is debated. In 1961, **Charnley** described the low-friction principle with the concept of a small femoral head. In 1972, results were reported by **Charnley** of 379 primary interventions performed in 3 years from 1962, and followed for up to 7 years. During this period, apart from infection, late failures were rare. Meanwhile, **Ring** described a complete replacement arthroplasty where both components were inherently stable and where cement was not required. Preliminary results were excellent.

Evaluation of Results – The Classics

Harris WH **Traumatic arthritis of the hip after dislocation and acetabular fractures; treatment by mould arthroplasty. An end-result study using a new method of result evaluation** J Bone Joint Surg [Am] 1969;51A:737–755

Merle D'Aubigne R, Postel M **Results of hip arthroplasty with acrylic prosthesis** J Bone Joint Surg [Am] 1954;36A:451–475

Harris first described his hip score for the assessment of mould arthroplasties in 1969. Points were awarded for pain, function as assessed by gait, absence of fixed deformity and range of motion. A maximum of 100 points was available. **Merle D'Aubigne** in 1954 described a system of assessment based on scores from 0–6 for each of pain, mobility and walking ability.

Callaghan JJ, Dysart SH, Savory CF, Hopkinson WJ **Assessing the results of hip replacement. A comparison of five different rating systems** J Bone Joint Surg [Br] 1990;72B:1008–1009

Brand RA, Pedersen D, Yoder SA **How definition of "loosening" affects the incidence of loose total hip reconstructions** Clin Orthop 1986;210:185–191

Galante J **Editorial: evaluation of the results of total hip replacement** J Bone Joint Surg [Am] 1990;72A:161–168

Johnston RC, Fitzgerald RH, Harris WH, Poss R, Müller ME, Sledge CB **Clinical and radiographic evaluation of total hip replacement** J Bone Joint Surg [Am] 1990;72A:161–168

Callaghan presented the results of 100 primary uncemented total hip replacements assessed by five different methods, including the modified Harris hip score and the Merle D'Aubigne rating. The Hospital for Special Surgery rating produced the most optimistic assessment and the Merle D'Aubigne rating the most pessimistic. There were significant differences between the results as assessed by the different systems. **Brand** noted that with the use of different definitions of "loosening", it was possible to produce a wide variation in the apparent rate of operative success. **Galante** set out the elements of the problem in an editorial, and **Johnston** produced a standardised nomenclature from which any desired hip score can be calculated.

Long-term Results of Cemented Arthroplasty

Wroblewski BM **Fifteen to 21-year results of the Charnley low-friction arthroplasty** Clin Orthop 1986;211:30–35

Cornell CN, Ranawat CS **Survivorship analysis of total hip replacements: results in a series of active patients who were less than 55 years old** J Bone Joint Surg [Am] 1986;68A:1430–1434

Halley DK, Wroblewski BM **Long-term results of low-friction arthroplasty in patients 30 years of age or younger** Clin Orthop 1986;211:43–50

Fowler JL Gie GA, Lee AJC, Ling RSM **Experience with the Exeter total hip replacement since 1970** Orthop Clin North Am 1988;19:477–489

Mulroy RD, Harris WH **The effect of improved cementing techniques on component loosening in total hip replacement** J Bone Joint Surg [Br] 1990; 72B:757–760

Wroblewski described the results of 116 Charnley arthroplasties performed 15–21 years previously. Clinical results were excellent (85% pain-free, 11% occasional discomfort). However, 22% of sockets migrated and this was statistically related to the depth of wear. It was stressed that these results were those from an early, unsophisticated technique. **Cornell** described the results of 101 primary total hip replacements in 85 patients who were less than 55 years old. Survivorship analysis was used to calculate a predicted cumulative rate of success for this series of total hip replacements over 10 years. This method of analysis of the data was chosen because it provided an expected durability of a total hip arthroplasty. Life-table calculations predicted that the survivorship of all the total hip replacements in this series would be 87% at 10 years of follow-up. This method of analysis provides a conservative estimation of rates of success and failure. **Halley** discussed the results of 49 Charnley arthroplasties performed in patients 30 years of age or younger at the time of surgery and followed for an average of 10 years. Only seven sockets, i.e. 14%, had failed, six with deficient bone stock at operation. Most of these patients suffered with general conditions such as rheumatoid arthritis, causing inbuilt restraints against overactivity. **Fowler** described excellent results at up to 17 years using a collarless femoral component which was designed to slide within the cement mantle. There were some early failures due to breakage of the component, but once this design fault had been eliminated, femoral failure due to aseptic loosening was extremely rare. **Mulroy** reported that by using improved cementing techniques, including a medullary plug and a cement gun, the rate of loosening of a collared femoral component could be reduced to 3% at 11 years. In contrast, despite improved cementation techniques, acetabular loosening was still 42% by this time.

Bone–Cement Interface

Ling RSM, Gie GA **Cement fixation for stemmed prostheses** In: Reynolds D, Freeman M, eds. Osteoarthritis in the young adult hip: options for surgical management. Edinburgh: Churchill Livingstone, 1989:183–204

Jasty M, Maloney WJ, Bragdon CP, Haire T, Harris WH **Histomorphometric studies of the long-term skeletal responses to well-fixed cemented femoral components** J Bone Joint Surg [Am] 1990;72A:1220–1231

Malcolm AJ **Pathology of long-standing cemented total hip replacement in Charnley's cases** J Bone Joint Surg [Br] 1988;70B:153

Ling reviews the role of acrylic bone cement with particular reference to its place in total hip replacement in the younger patient. Its long-term acceptability to local skeletal tissue and the host as a whole are discussed. The importance of achieving direct contact between cement and living bone is emphasised, and methods for optimising contact and improving cement properties are illustrated. **Jasty** studied femora obtained at autopsy from patients who had previously had a cemented total hip replacement. The time between implantation and autopsy was between 40 months and 17.5 years. Clinically and radiographically the prostheses had been functioning well prior to death and had shown no signs of loosening. Histological examination showed that host bone was intimately and directly opposed to the cement with a dense shell of substantial new bone around the cement mantle which resembled a new cortex and which was attached to the outer cortex by trabecular struts. The cemented femoral components were well tolerated by the skeleton, and fibrous tissue had rarely formed at the femoral cement–bone interface. **Malcolm** reported on 78 total hip replacement specimens retrieved from 61 patients after death. They had been inserted by the late Sir John Charnley, a mean of 17 years previously, and all had excellent clinical results. The study showed that long-term cement implantation could produce a stable tissue integration. Trabecular microfractures were one cause of late loosening. Tissue reaction to wear particles was likely to be a major contributory factor in loosening of the acetabular cup.

Osseointegration

Albrektsson T, Albrektsson B **Osseointegration of bone implants – a review of an alternative mode of fixation** Acta Orthop Scand 1987;78:567–577

Linder L, Carlsson A, Marsal L, Bjursten LM, Branemark PI **Clinical aspects of osseointegration in joint replacement: a histological study of titanium implants** J Bone Joint Surg [Br] 1988;70B:550–555

Haddad RJ, Cook SD, Thomas KA **Current concepts review: biological fixation of porous coated implants** J Bone Joint Surg [Am] 1987;69A:1459–1466

Albrektsson provides a review of the subject. **Linder** demonstrated that it was possible to produce osseointegration around a titanium implant in humans, even in the presence of rheumatoid arthritis. **Haddad** reviewed the situation with particular reference to total joint replacements in humans.

Uncemented Arthroplasty

Freeman MAR **The fixation of prostheses without cement** In: Catterall A, ed. Recent advances in orthopaedics 5. London: Churchill Livingstone, 1987: 1–17

Ring PA **Press-fit prostheses: clinical experience** In: Reynolds D, Freeman MAR, eds. Osteoarthritis of the young adult hip. London: Churchill Livingstone, 1989:220–232

Nunn D **The Ring uncemented plastic-on-metal total hip replacement** J Bone Joint Surg [Br] 1988;70B:40–44

Callaghan JJ, Dysart SH, Savory CG. **The uncemented porous-coated anatomic total hip prosthesis: 2-year results of a prospective consecutive series** J Bone Joint Surg [Am] 1988;70A:337–346

Engh CA, Bobyn JD, Glassman AH. **Porous coated hip replacement: the factors governing bone ingrowth, stress shielding, and clinical results** J Bone Joint Surg [Br] 1987;69B:45–55

Engh CA, Griffin WL, Marx CL **Cementless acetabular components** J Bone Joint Surg [Br] 1990;72B:53–59

Maloney WJ, Harris WH **Comparison of a hybrid with an uncemented total hip replacement** J Bone Joint Surg [Am] 1990; 72A:1349–1352

Freeman discusses the concept of uncemented fixation of prostheses. Prostheses are divided into press-fit and bone-ingrowth types. The requirements for a stable press-fit are suggested to be the elimination of interfacial shear and tension and the reduction of compression stresses to below the failure strength of the materials. The conditions necessary for tissue ingrowth to occur are explored and the evidence for bony ingrowth is summarised. The lack of long-term data for loosening rates for porous surfaces is emphasised. **Ring** discusses the design and technique of insertion of his prosthesis. The results of 172 replacements performed in young patients for osteoarthritis are presented; 106 prostheses were of a metal-on-metal type and were followed for between 7 and 17 years. Sixty-six replacements were metal-on-plastic and follow-up was for between 1 and 6 years. The merits and disadvantages of uncemented joint replacement are debated: thigh pain and "start-up" pain are common, but diminish with time. Minor bone defects on the acetabular side may resolve spontaneously and femoral revision is relatively easy if the failure is mechanical. **Nunn** reviewed the results of 1488 Ring prostheses with a follow up of 2–7 years. There was an excellent clinical result in 93% overall and in 87% of those cases which had been followed for more than 5 years. **Callaghan** reported the 2-year results of 50 uncemented prostheses. There was persistent thigh pain in 8 cases and a moderate or severe limp in 13 patients. There was a high incidence of radiodense lines around the femoral component, the significance of which was unclear. A significant number of components showed loss of the porous coating. **Engh** (1989) reviewed the results of 307 uncemented total hip replacement procedures with particular reference to aspects of the femoral component which might affect bone ingrowth, stress shielding and the clinical result. The incidence of both pain and limp was much lower when there was either a press-fit or evidence of bone ingrowth. Bone ingrowth appeared to give better results than fibrous tissue fixation. **Engh** (1990) compared the results of 415 total hip replacements using an uncemented acetabular component of either a porous-ingrowth or smooth-threaded design. After a mean follow-up of 4.8 years, none of the porous-ingrowth cups showed any sign of failure, whereas after a mean of 3.7 years, 21% of patients with a threaded cup demonstrated radiographic signs of failure and 25% had clinical symptoms. **Maloney** reported the short-term results of a hybrid hip replacement in which an uncemented acetabular component and a cemented femoral component were used, comparing this prosthesis with a completely uncemented prosthesis. After a short follow-up (3 years), the results of the hybrid replacement were superior.

Resurfacing

Amstutz HC **Recent advances in total hip resurfacing** In: McKibbin B, ed. Recent advances in orthopaedics 4. Edinburgh: Churchill Livingstone 1983: 155–177

Amstutz HC, Thomas BJ, Jinnah R, Kim W, Grogan T, Yale C **Treatment of primary osteoarthritis of the hip: a comparison of total joint and surface replacement arthroplasty** J Bone Joint Surg [Am] 1984;66A:228–241

Freeman MAR **The complications of double-cup replacement of the hip** In: Ling RSM, ed. Complications of total hip replacement. Edinburgh: Churchill Livingstone, 1984:172–200

Howie DW, Campbell D, McGee M, Cornish BL **Wagner resurfacing hip arthroplasty. The results of 100 consecutive arthroplasties after 8–10 years** J Bone Joint Surg [Am] 1990;72A:708–714

Amstutz (1983) discussed the development of the Tharies surface replacement and the indications for its use. The surgical technique is described and the results of the first 350 cases reported. There was good pain relief, enhanced joint stability and a low incidence of infection. Later, **Amstutz** (1984) compared the results of a conventional total hip replacement with those of a Tharies surface replacement. The surface replacements were performed on a younger and more active group of patients. There was no difference in the results between the two groups in terms of pain relief, walking ability and movement. An important radiolucent line was noted in 57% of the surface replacements at 3 years compared to a 38% incidence following a total hip replacement at 4 years. **Freeman** discussed the complications that follow surface replacement of the hip. Most were due to errors both in the earlier designs of the prostheses and in technique. The procedure should be restricted to a small number of surgeons and precise indications must be observed in its use. **Howie** studied 100 consecutive Wagner resurfacing hip arthroplasties in 93 patients. The rate of survival of the arthroplasty was 70% at 5 years but only 40% at 8 years. The major cause of failure was aseptic loosening of the acetabular or femoral component or both. Fracture of the neck of the femur occurred in three hips. They conclude that studies of new prosthetic designs of resurfacing arthroplasty must be continued for at least 8 years.

Migration

Loudon JR, Charnley J **Subsidence of the femoral prosthesis in total hip replacement in relation to the design of the stem** J Bone Joint Surg [Br] 1980; 62B:450–453

Mjoberg B, Selvik G, Hansson LI, Rosenqvist R, Onnerfalt R **Mechanical loosening of total hip prostheses: a radiographic and roentgen stereophotogrammetric study** J Bone Joint Surg [Br] 1986;68B:770–774

Amstutz HC, Ouzounion T, Grauer T, Flink C, Kirkpatrick J, Bassett L **The grid radiograph: a simple technique for consistent high resolution visualisation of the hip** J Bone Joint Surg [Am] 1986;68A:1052–1056

Louden examined the influence of an alteration in the design of femoral stem on subsidence. He demonstrated that alteration of the stem design can reduce the rate of subsidence and the incidence of cement fractures. Measurements were performed using a ruler. **Mjoberg** described the technique of roentgen stereophotogrammetry, in which tantalum markers were inserted in the region of the femoral and acetabular components. Using simultaneous orthogonal radiographs, it was possible to measure subsidence to a high degree of accuracy. Minor degrees of subsidence commonly occurred. **Amstutz** described a technique for assessing migration accurately on a standardised radiograph.

Aseptic Loosening

Evans EM, Freeman MAR, Miller AJ, Vernon-Roberts B **Metal sensitivity as a cause of bone necrosis and loosening of the prosthesis in total joint replacement** J Bone Joint Surg [Br] 1974;56B:626–642

Goldring SR, Schiller AL, Roelke M, Rourke CM, O'Neill DA, Harris WH **The synovial-like membrane at the bone–cement interface in loose total hip replacements and its proposed role in bone lysis** J Bone Joint Surg [Am] 1983; 65A:575–584

Linder L, Lindberg L, Carlsson A **Aseptic loosening of hip prostheses: a histologic and enzyme histochemical study** Clin Orthop 1983;175:93–104

Jones LC, Hungerford DS **Cement disease** Clin Orthop 1987;225:192–206

Howie DW, Vernon-Roberts B, Oakeshot R, Manthey B **A rat model of resorption of bone at the cement–bone interface in the presence of polyethylene wear particles** J Bone Joint Surg [Am] 1988;70A:257–263

Lombardi A V, Mallory TH, Vaughan BK, Drouillard P **Aseptic loosening in total hip arthroplasty secondary to osteolysis induced by wear debris from titanium alloy modular femoral heads** J Bone Joint Surg [Am] 1989;71A: 1337–1342

Lennox DW, Schofield BH, McDonald DF, Riley LH **A histological comparison of aseptic loosening of cemented, press-fit and biologic-ingrowth prostheses** Clin Orthop 1987;225:171–191

Maloney WJ, Jasty M, Rosenberg A, Harris WH **Bone lysis in well-fixed cemented femoral components** J Bone Joint Surg [Br] 1990;72B:966–970

Anthony PP, Gie GA, Howie CR, Ling RSM **Localized endosteal bone lysis in relation to the femoral components of cemented total hip arthroplasties** J Bone Joint Surg [Br] 1990;72B:971–979

Santavirta S, Hoikka V, Eskola A, Konttinen YT, Paavilainen T, Tallroth K **Aggressive granulomatosis lesions in cementless total hip arthroplasty** J Bone Joint Surg [Br] 1990;72B:980–984

Evans suggested that aseptic loosening of a total joint prosthesis could be due to a hypersensitivity reaction to metal ions. **Goldring** showed that the pseudocapsule around a total hip replacement which had loosened aseptically had a well-defined structure resembling a synovial lining. The cells from this membrane had the capacity to produce prostaglandin E_2 and collagenase. **Linder** investigated the membrane histologically, and using enzyme histochemistry concluded that loosening was primarily a mechanical event. **Jones** suggested that hypersensitivity to methylmethacrylate cement might be implicated in loosening. **Howie** demonstrated that polyethylene wear debris was able to induce an appearance similar to aseptic loosening in a rat model using cement; in the absence of polyethylene wear particles a stable bone–cement interface was formed. **Lombardi** suggested that titanium wear debris may produce localised osteolysis. **Lennox** compared the histological appearance of membranes from aseptically loose cemented and uncemented prostheses. Although the membranes were similar, the uncemented prosthesis membrane was less aggressive. **Maloney** investigated focal osteolysis adjacent to well-fixed, cemented femoral implants. In the majority of cases, the lucency corresponded to an area of deficient cement; and cement fractures were shown in three cases at postmortem. The rate of progression of the area of lysis was variable, but in one case frank loosening developed. **Anthony** described four cases where osteolysis developed in relation to otherwise well-fixed femoral components. In each case the area of lysis was related to a local defect in the cement mantle surrounding the stem. Through the space between the stem and the cement, transport of wear debris from the joint could occur directly to the endosteal surface of the bone, so giving rise to the lysis. **Santavirta** reported five cases where lytic lesions similar to those previously described in relation to cemented prostheses occurred in association with uncemented prostheses. The initiating factor appeared to be polythene wear debris from the acetabular cup.

Total Hip Arthroplasty in Special Groups

Congenital Dislocation of the Hip

Harris WH **Total hip replacement for osteoarthritis secondary to congenital dysplasia or congenital dislocation of the hip** Int Orthop 1978;2:127–138

Woolson ST, Harris WH **Complex total hip replacement for dysplastic or hypoplastic hips using miniature or microminiature components** J Bone Joint Surg [Am] 1983;65A:1099–1108

Paavilainen T, Hoikka V, Solonen KA **Cementless total replacement for severely dysplastic or dislocated hips** J Bone Joint Surg [Br] 1990;72B: 205–211

Harris divided dysplastic hips into three groups, those with mild anatomical deformity; those with moderate and those with severe acetabular deficiency requiring bone grafting. The pitfalls and solutions are discussed,with helpful illustrations. **Woolson** described the use of miniature custom-made femoral components in 69 cases. The importance of preoperative planning to determine the appropriate size of the components is stressed; a full complement of miniature femoral and acetabular components is necessary. Results were gratifying despite the technical difficulties encountered. **Paavilainen** reported early results of 100 cementless total hip replacements in 52 severely dysplastic and 48 totally dislocated hips. Techniques for dealing with the problems of acetabular insufficiency and proximal femoral abnormalities are described. Although the complication rates were high, the results were generally good.

Paget's Disease

McDonald DJ, Sim FH **Total hip arthroplasty in Paget's disease – a follow-up note** J Bone Joint Surg [Am] 1987;69A:766–772

McDonald discussed experience with total hip arthroplasty in 91 hips. Loosening occurs more commonly in patients with Paget's disease; however, the overall results were good or excellent in 74%. Thus cemented total hip replacement remains an acceptable form of treatment.

Rheumatoid Arthritis

Ranawat CS **Surgery for rheumatoid arthritis. 2: Lower limb; 1: Surgery of the hip** Curr Orthop 1989; 3(3):146–149

Poss R, Maloney JP, Ewald FC, Thomas WH, Batte NJ, Hartness C, Sledge C **Six to eleven-year results of total hip arthroplasty in rheumatoid arthritis** Clin Orthop 1984;182:109–116

Ranawat reviewed the problems of surgery of the hip in rheumatoid arthritis, with emphasis on protrusio acetabuli, fibrous or bony ankylosis, and avascular necrosis. Osteotomy and arthrodesis have no place in the management of hip disease in rheumatoid patients. Cemented total hip replacement is the treatment of choice; however there are few reports of long-term results. The results of 138 total hip arthroplasties were reviewed by **Poss** 7 years after operation. Ninety-six per cent were clinically improved but their functional requirements were less. Mechanical loosening was likely with time.

Juvenile Arthritis

Ruddlesdin C, Ansell BM, Arden GP, Swann M **Total hip replacement in children with juvenile chronic arthritis** J Bone Joint Surg [Br] 1986;68B: 218–222

The results of 75 total hip replacements are reported by **Ruddlesdin** with a mean follow-up of 5 years. Careful selection is essential, and in these cases the results obtained were gratifying. Assessment by a rheumatologist is essential.

Ankylosing Spondylitis

Williams E, Taylor AR, Arden GP, Edwards DH **Arthroplasty of the hip in ankylosing spondylitis** J Bone Joint Surg [Br] 1977;59B:393–397

Kilgus DJ, Namba RS, Govek JE, Cracchiolo A, Amstutz HC **Total hip replacement for patients who have ankylosing spondylitis** J Bone Joint Surg [Am] 1990;72A:834–839

Williams in 1977 provided a useful reference on the subject of hip arthroplasty in ankylosing spondylitis. These patients need the operation at a younger age than osteoarthritic cases. Seventy-three per cent of 86 hips were graded excellent or good 10 years after surgery. The most troublesome problem was recurrence of ankylosis, with pain and periarticular ossification. **Kilgus** reported the results of 53 total hip replacement procedures in 31 patients after an average follow-up of 6.3 years. Cemented hip replacements gave good long-term results in this population group.

Femoral Osteotomy

Benke GJ, Baker AS, Dounis E **Total hip replacement after upper femoral osteotomy: a clinical review** J Bone Joint Surg [Br] 1982;64B:570–571

Benke in 1982 reviewed the results of 105 total hip replacement patients who had undergone previous upper femoral osteotomy for osteoarthritis. At 5 years 90% had a satisfactory result. The infection rate was 8.6%. Occasional surgical difficulties were encountered. It was concluded that upper femoral osteotomy does not seriously prejudice the outcome of a subsequent total hip replacement.

Arthrodesis

Brewster RC, Coventry MB, Johnson EW **Conversion of the arthrodesed hip to a total hip arthroplasty** J Bone Joint Surg [Am] 1975;57A:27–30

Hardinge K, Williams D, Etienne A, MacKenzie D, Charnley J **Conversion of fused hips to low-friction arthroplasty** J Bone Joint Surg [Br] 1977;59B: 385–392

Brewster described experience where a total hip arthroplasty was performed in 33 patients who had previously undergone surgical attempts at arthrodesis. Thirty-one patients had a satisfactory functional result after 1–3.5 years. **Hardinge** discussed the results of 54 hips converted to low-friction arthroplasty in a 10-year period and reviewed after 1–11 years. In many, malposition of the arthrodesis had led to degenerative changes in the opposite hip, the lumbar spine or the knee, often with severe loss of function due to pain. Total replacement gave useful relief of pain and improved function, although the range of movement obtained was not as good as in primary replacement. An outstanding feature was the correction of inequality of leg length. Surgical techniques are described in detail.

Acetabular Deficiency

Gerber SD, Harris WH **Femoral head autografting to augment acetabular deficiency in patients requiring total hip replacement: A minimum 5-year and average 7-year follow-up study** J Bone Joint Surg [Am] 1986;68A: 1241–1248

Jasty M, Harris WH **Salvage total hip reconstruction in patients with major acetabular bone loss** J Bone Joint Surg [Br] 1990;72B:63–67

Gerber reviewed the results of 47 hip replacements in patients with dysplastic acetabulae, in which the femoral head was used as an augmentation autograft. All united but resorption occurred in a high percentage. There was a high incidence of complications. In patients who do not have autograft available, allograft femoral heads can be used. **Jasty** evaluated 30 such hip reconstructions. All the allografts united, but the acetabular loosening rate rose from 0 at 4 years to 32% at 6 years. Allografts provide only a short-term solution in these difficult cases.

Sickle-cell Disease

Clarke HJ, Jinnah RH, Brooker AF, Michaelson JD **Total replacement of the hip for avascular necrosis in sickle-cell disease** J Bone Joint Surg [Br] 1989; 71B:465–470

Clarke discussed the particular problems of sickle-cell anaemia with avascular necrosis in 27 patients. There were important medical problems. Most patients required transfusion before surgery, which prevented postoperative sickle-cell crises. In some, operation revealed sclerotic bone with obliteration of the femoral canal. There was also a high morbidity due to loosening in both cemented and uncemented prostheses. The paper serves as a very useful reminder of the general medical problems in the treatment of patients with sickle-cell disease.

Following Infection

Cherney DL, Amstutz HC **Total hip replacement in the previously septic hip** J Bone Joint Surg [Am] 1983;65A:1256–1265

Cherney discussed total hip replacement performed in either one or two stages in 33 hips with active sepsis. Thirty-three (70%) revealed no signs of infection at 3–9 years after prosthetic replacement. The success rate was higher when the original organism was Gram-positive rather than Gram-negative. In patients with a successful total hip replacement, function was better than those with a Girdlestone procedure.

Following Tuberculosis of the Hip

Hardinge K, Williams D, Etienne A, MacKenzie D, Charnley J **Conversion of fused hips to low-friction arthroplasty** J Bone Joint Surg [Br] 1977;59B: 385–392

Tuli SM, Mukherjee SK **Excision arthroplasty for tuberculosis and pyogenic arthritis of the hip** J Bone Joint Surg [Br] 1981;63B:29–32

Eskola A, Santavirta S, Konttinen YT, Tallroth K, Hoikka V, Lindholm ST **Cementless total replacement for old tuberculosis of the hip** J Bone Joint Surg [Br] 1988;70B:603–606

Kim Y-H, Han D-Y, Park B-M **Total hip arthroplasty for tuberculous coxarthrosis** J Bone Joint Surg [Am] 1987;69A:718–727

Hardinge has narrated experience with the conversion of fused hips to low-friction arthroplasty. In some of the 54 hips, the original cause was tuberculous infection in childhood. Total replacement gave useful relief of pain and improved function, with correction of inequality of leg length. **Tuli** discussed the results for 30 patients with chronic pyogenic or tuberculous arthritis of the hip treated by excision arthroplasty. It was stressed that the functional needs of patients in India differ from those in the affluent countries. Excision arthroplasty is considered a sound operation to restore the ability to squat and sit cross-legged. **Eskola** reported the results of cementless total joint replacement in 18 patients in Finland with old tuberculosis of the hip performed, on average, 34 years after infection. Only 7 of the patients had antituberculous drugs during or after the operation. There was a high percentage of excellent or good results, with no reactivation of tuberculosis. **Kim** discussed experience with 44 total hip prostheses in Korea. The interval between active disease and total hip arthroplasty ranged from 3 months to 45 years. Three-quarters had a good result at 4 years follow-up, but 6 patients had reactivation of the disease controlled satisfactorily by chemotherapy alone or debridement of sinus tracks without removal of the prosthesis. Recurrence was more likely in those who had inactive disease for less than 10 years. Total hip arthroplasty was considered a safe procedure whether the infection was quiescent, or somewhat, but not aggressively, active.

Complications

Vascular and Neurological Complications

Ratliff AHC **Vascular and Neurological complications** In: Ling RSM, ed. Complications of total hip replacement. Edinburgh: Churchill Livingstone, 1984:18–29

Ratliff discussed the wide variety of causes that can produce major vascular and neurological complications following total hip replacement, based on a collected series of cases. It was concluded that most, if not all, of these complications can be prevented with meticulous attention to detail when performing this operation.

Fractures of the Femur

Cook PH, Newman JH **Fractures of the femur in relation to cemented hip prostheses** J Bone Joint Surg [Br] 1988;70B:386–389

Cook reviewed the results of treatment of 75 fractures of the proximal femoral shaft in the presence of a cemented femoral prosthesis. Four types of fracture were described. Comminuted fractures round the implant required early revision, whilst spiral fractures in this region may be treated conservatively or by operation. Transverse fractures at the level of the tip of the prosthesis are difficult to manage and may require open reduction and internal fixation. The choice of treatment in individual cases may be influenced by the presence of infection or gross destruction of bone.

Infection – Prevention

Charnley J **A clean-air operating enclosure** Clin Orthop 1986;211:4–9

Waugh W **Clean air against infection** In: Waugh W, ed. John Charnley: The man and the hip. London: Springer-Verlag, 1989

Lidwell OM, Lowbury EJL, Whyte W, Blowers R, Stanley SJ, Lowe D **Effect of ultra-clean air in operating rooms on deep sepsis in the joint after total hip or knee replacement: a randomised study** Br Med J 1982;285:10–14

Trippel SB **Current concepts review: antibiotic-impregnated cement in total joint arthroplasty** J Bone Joint Surg [Am] 1986;68A:1297–1302

Laurence M **Clean air and the use of antibiotics in surgery** In: Catterall A, ed. Recent advances in orthopaedics 5. London: Churchill Livingstone, 1987: 153–163

Thyne GM, Ferguson JW **Antibiotic prophylaxis during dental treatment in patients with prosthetic joints** J Bone Joint Surg [Br] 1990;72B:191–194

The consequences of deep infection around a joint replacement are disastrous, and Charnley faced this problem when he began carrying out arthroplasties in 1960. In a classic article, (originally published in 1964) **Charnley** conceived the idea of reducing the number of bacteria suspended in the air in the operating room by filtration and dilution. **Waugh** described Charnley's studies on bacterial contamination in the operating theatre and the development of a clean-air operating enclosure with the use of body exhaust gown. An MRC study group was created to evaluate the benefit of clean air systems. A large prospective series was analysed. **Lidwell** provided evidence that the cleanliness of the air had a significant effect on the incidence of deep infection. **Trippel** debated the use of antibiotic-impregnated cement. Because of the low rates of infection now routinely achieved, it was not possible to demonstrate an additional lowering of the infection rate. He therefore concluded that its use was not justified for routine cases. **Laurence** considered that the evidence is now incontrovertible that preoperative antibiotics substantially reduce the risk of deep joint sepsis. Errors of surgical technique remain the major hazards. Ordinary surgical standards are not adequate when foreign implants are introduced. Absolute sterility remains a theoretical goal; but there is still a risk of haematogenous invasion threatening a small percentage of cases.

Thyne debates the role of prophylactic antimicrobial therapy to cover dental procedures in patients who have undergone total joint replacement. There is no convincing published evidence to support a general policy of antibiotic prophylaxis in these circumstances. Patients with rheumatoid arthritis, reoperated hips and those on steroids or immunosuppressive agents, constitute a high-risk group and in these patients prophylaxis may be justified. Significant bacteraemias of dental origin occur mainly in patients with advanced periodontal disease or generalised dental sepsis. These patients should be identified and treated prior to joint replacement.

Infection – Treatment

Buchholz HW, Elson RA, Engelbrecht E, Loden Kamper H, Rottger J, Siegel A **Management of deep infection of total hip replacement** J Bone Joint Surg [Br] 1981;63B:342–353

Gustilo RB, Leagogo LAC **Management of infected total hip replacement** In: Gustilo RB, ed. Orthopaedic infection: diagnosis and treatment. Philadelphia: WB Saunders, 1989

With an experience of 583 patients, **Buchholz** recommended an exchange operation as the treatment of choice for most deep infections. This revision arthroplasty comprises, in one stage, excision of soft tissue, removal of implant and cement and replacement with an implant using cement loaded with an appropriate antibiotic. More recently, systemic antibiotics have also been employed. During the period before systemic antibiotics were used, a 77% success rate was achieved. There was a significant morbidity; these operations are major procedures, often in elderly patients who have suffered previous operations and infection. Failure was associated with infection with certain organisms, delay in operation, and inadequate amounts of antibiotic in the cement. The decision as to whether subsequent exchange operations should be carried out after failure of the first attempt is difficult, but reoperation was successful in 90% of cases. **Gustilo** described an algorithm for treatment of an infected total hip replacement. He divided cases into three groups: acute sepsis, delayed infection and chronic infection. A scheme is offered for the management of each group. He does not recommend immediate exchange arthroplasty except in elderly patients who cannot withstand another operation when the organism is less virulent. Improved results have been obtained with delayed exchange. Indications for resection arthroplasty are debated; they include those with virulent resistant organisms in unhealthy scarred tissue and with severe bone loss.

Thromboembolism

Sikorski JM **Thromboembolic complications** In: Ling RSM ed. Complications of total hip replacement. Edinburgh: Churchill Livingstone, 1984:58–81

Hull RD, Raskob GE **Current concepts review: prophylaxis of venous thromboembolic disease following hip and knee surgery** J Bone Joint Surg [Am] 1986;68A:146–150

Planes A, Vochelle N, Fagola M **Total hip replacement and deep vein thrombosis** J Bone Joint Surg [Br] 1990;72B:9–13

Woolson ST, McCoy DW, Stanford JW, Maloney WJ, Watt M, Cahill PD **B-mode ultrasound scanning in the detection of proximal venous thrombosis after total hip replacement** J Bone Joint Surg [Am] 1990;72A:983–987

Turpie AGG **Enoxaparin prophylaxis in elective hip surgery** Acta Chir Scand Suppl 1990;556:103–107

Thromboembolism is a large subject and numerous studies have shown clotting in the calf or thigh veins in up to 50% of patients after elective hip surgery. Diagnosis, and more particularly, prophylaxis remain controversial. **Sikorski** discussed the methods of diagnosis, the natural history of deep vein thrombosis, prophylaxis and treatment. He concluded that effective prophylaxis is limited to the avoidance of high-risk factors when feasible, and that anticoagulants seem ineffective and potentially hazardous. **Hull** stressed the inaccuracy of clinical diagnosis and the difficulty of obtaining studies which compare a method of prophylaxis with a concurrent control group. The use of aspirin, heparin, intermittent pneumatic compression and combined modalities are debated. Three approaches to primary prophylaxis are considered to be effective and recommended. They entail the use of (a) warfarin, (b) adjusted-dose subcutaneous heparin, or (c) intermittent pneumatic compression and dextran. Hull concluded that any of these approaches would be reasonable for elective surgery on the hip. **Planes** reported the results of bilateral venography in 745 consecutive total hip replacement patients, all of whom received heparin prophylaxis. Of these, 81 showed evidence of recent deep vein thrombosis. Twenty-three were distal, 44 isolated proximal, and 14 involved both segments. Although the number of thromboses had been reduced by heparin, the drug was less effective at reducing proximal thromboses. In a cadaver study, kinking or folding of the proximal femoral vein was shown to occur during femoral preparation. **Woolson** undertook a prospective comparison of the utility of B-mode ultrasound scanning and ascending venography following total hip replacement in 143 patients. Ultrasound scanning was a sensitive and specific method for diagnosing proximal thromboses. **Turpie** reported a randomised double-blind placebo-controlled study of the efficacy of 30 mg of low molecular weight heparin given subcutaneously twice daily, in the prevention of thrombosis. Deep venous thrombosis occurred in 6 of 50 treated patients compared with 21 controls, while proximal segment thromboses were reduced from 10 in the control group to 2. Treatment was not associated with bleeding complications.

Stem Breakage

Galante JO **Current concepts review: causes of fractures of the femoral component in total hip replacement** J Bone Joint Surg [Am] 1980;62A: 670–673

Lee AJC, Ling RSM **Stem breakage** In: Ling RSM, ed. Complications of total hip replacement. London: Churchill Livingstone, 1984:146–171

Galante stated that fractures of the femoral stem component are usually in the middle third; the population at risk is the heavy male. There is a high incidence of varus with loosening and lack of support at the calcar femorale. **Lee** notes that the incidence of stem breakage is now low. By an appropriate combination of materials, design and technique, the problem may be reduced. There is a close relationship between the factors that lead to breakage and those that lead to loosening.

Dislocation

Ali Khan MA, Brakenbury PH, Reynolds ISR **Dislocation following total hip replacement** J Bone Joint Surg [Br] 1981;63B:214–218

Hamblen DL **Dislocation**. In: Ling RSM, ed. Complications of total hip replacement. Edinburgh: Churchill Livingstone, 1984:82–90

In a study of 6774 arthroplasties from three centres, **Ali Khan** divided dislocations into early and late occurrences; the arbitrary division was 5 weeks after surgery. Patients at special risk included those who were confused or those undergoing revision procedures. The most common surgical error was placing the acetabular cup too vertically or too anteverted; a less common fault was placing the femoral component too anteverted. Seventy-eight per cent of 142 dislocations eventually obtained stability. **Hamblen** discussed the clinical features, prevention and treatment of dislocation after hip replacement. Factors contributing to instability and dislocation are the design of the implant, the technique of insertion and the stability of the soft tissues. Technical errors, particularly malalignment of the components, account for the majority of dislocations. A very aged patient is especially at risk.

Related to Trochanteric Osteotomy

Hamblen DL **Complications of trochanteric osteotomy** In: Ling RSM, ed. Complications of total hip replacement. Edinburgh: Churchill Livingstone, 1984: 91–99

Wroblewski BM, Shelley P **Reattachment of the greater trochanter after hip replacement** J Bone Joint Surg [Br] 1985;67B:736–740

One of the most controversial topics since the introduction of the operation of total hip replacement has been the need to detach the great trochanter. The advantages and disadvantages of trochanteric osteotomy are marshalled by **Hamblen**. The major complications of trochanteric osteotomy relate to defective fixation and subsequent non-union. **Wroblewski** described a method of performing a biplanar trochanteric osteotomy with a Gigli saw, which had been tested in 431 cases. The results of three methods of trochanteric reattachment are analysed. The optimal method involved a double crossover wire with a compression spring, which was successful in a high percentage of cases.

Ectopic Ossification – The Classic

Brooker AF, Bowerman JW, Robinson RA, Riley LH Jr **Ectopic ossification following total hip replacement: incidence and a method of classification** J Bone Joint Surg [Am] 1973;55A:1629–1632

Brooker noted ectopic bone formation following 21% of 100 consecutive total hip arthroplasty procedures. The ossification did not impair the clinical result. A classification of the severity of ossification is presented.

Ayers DC, Evarts CM, Parkinson JR **The prevention of heterotopic ossification in high-risk patients by low-dose radiation therapy after total hip arthroplasty** J Bone Joint Surg [Am] 1986;68A:1423–1430

Konski A, Pellegrini V, Poulter C, De Vanny J, Rosier R, Evarts CM, Hanzler M, Rubin P **Randomized trial comparing single-dose versus fractionated irradiation for prevention of heterotopic bone: a preliminary report** Int J Radiat Oncol Biol Phys 1989; 18:1139–1142

Schmidt SA, Kjaersgaard-Andersen P, Pedersen NW, Kristensen SK, Pedersen P, Nielsen JB **The use of indomethacin to prevent the formation of heterotopic bone after total hip replacement. A random, double-blind clinical trial** J Bone Joint Surg [Am] 1988;70A:834–838

Patients at high risk for heterotopic ossification include those with hypertrophic osteoarthritis, with new bone formation after previous arthroplasty, and those with post-traumatic arthritis. **Ayers** showed that 1000 rads of radiation administered over a period of 5 days was effective in the prevention of heterotopic ossification. **Konski** reported the preliminary results of a prospective study comparing a single dose of 800 rads with a 1000-rad multidose regimen. The lower dose was equally efficacious. **Schmidt** demonstrated that indomethacin was also effective in the prevention of heterotopic ossification.

Revision Arthroplasty

Clinical Studies – Cemented

Pellicci PM, Wilson PD, Sledge CB, Salvati EA, Ranawat CS, Poss R, Callaghan JJ **Long-term results of revision total hip replacement: a follow-up report** J Bone Joint Surg [Am] 1985;67A:513–516

Kavanagh BF, Ilstrup DM, Fitzgerald RH **Revision total hip arthroplasty** J Bone Joint Surg [Am] 1985;67A:517–526

Maiti RK, Schüller HM, Besselaar PP, Haashoot P **Results of revision hip arthroplasty with cement. A 5–14-year follow-up study** J Bone Joint Surg [Am] 1990;72A:346–354

Engelbrecht DJ, Weber FA, Sweet MBE, Jakim I **Long-term results of revision total hip arthroplasty** J Bone Joint Surg [Br] 1990;72B:41–45

The results of revision arthroplasty are difficult to interpret since methods of assessment are variable. **Pellicci** described the results in 99 patients 8 years after operation. Mechanical failure (loosening and fracture) occurred in 29%. **Kavanagh** reported results after a 4-year follow-up and suggested that there was probable loosening in 25% of the acetabular components. **Maiti** reviewed the results of 60 revision procedures after between 5 and 14 years. There had been two infections and four additional revisions for aseptic failure. There were signs of loosening in 10 cups and 16 femoral stems. Survivorship analysis of a group of 80 cases suggested an 85% 14-year survival. **Engelbrecht** reported the results of 138 revision procedures followed for an average of 7.4 years. There had been 14 reoperations for mechanical failure and three for sepsis. Better results were found when both components were replaced. There were good-to-excellent Mayo hip scores in 62% and 86% were pain-free. There was a high incidence of radiographic loosening.

Clinical Studies – Uncemented

Hungerford DS, Jones LC **The rationale of cementless revision of cemented arthroplasty failures** Clin Orthop 1988;235:12–24

Engh CA, Glassman AH, Griffin WL, Mayer JG **Results of cementless revision for failed cemented total hip arthoplasty** Clin Orthop 1988;235: 91–110

Eskola A, Santavirta S, Konttinen YT, Hoikka V, Tallroth K, Lindholm TS **Cementless revision of aggressive granulomatous lesions in hip replacements** J Bone Joint Surg [Br] 1990;72B:212–216

Hungerford proposed cementless revision of a failed cemented total hip replacement in order to improve deficient bone stock. **Engh** discussed his experience with 160 revision procedures using a cementless porous-ingrowth prosthesis, after a mean follow-up of 4.4 years. Implant fixation was graded as bone ingrowth, stable fibrous encapsulation, questionable with signs of impending instability or definitely unstable with implant migration, indicative of the need for further revision. The operations were graded according to the severity of pre-existing bone stock damage, and this was a factor in predicting the success of the revision. **Eskola** reported the results of revision of cemented hip replacements in which failure had been accompanied by the formation of aggressive granulomatous lesions, with an uncemented prosthesis. Sixteen cases are discussed, with a mean follow-up of 3.5 years. There were no recurrences.

Bone Grafting

McGann W, Mankin HJ, Harris WH **Massive allografting for severe failed total hip replacement** J Bone Joint Surg [Am] 1986;68A:4–12

Brien WW, Bruce WJ, Salvati EA, Wilson PD, Pellicci PM **Acetabular reconstruction with a bipolar prosthesis and morseled bone grafts** J Bone Joint Surg [Am] 1990;72A:1230–1235

Salvage of a failed total hip replacement with severe loss of bone stock provides a considerable challenge. **McGann** reported five cases where femoral bone stock was improved with large, frozen osteoarticular allografts from a bone bank. The grafts are not viable but provide a structural continuity which aids functional recovery. Severe acetabular deficiency can be overcome using femoral head autografts to support the acetabulum. **Brien** discussed the results of 18 acetabular reconstructions in which major defects had been treated by the use of a smooth bipolar prosthesis and impacted morcellized bone graft. In 11 cases the procedure had failed. In six there was complete resorption of the graft and in three cases there was infection. An improved acetabular bone structure was maintained in only four cases.

Excision Arthroplasty

Haw CS, Gray DH **Excision arthroplasty of the hip** J Bone Joint Surg [Br] 1976;58B:44–47

Clegg J **The results of the pseudarthrosis after removal of an infected total hip prosthesis** J Bone Joint Surg [Br] 1977;59B:298–301

Hamblen DL, Fisher WD **Excision arthroplasty as a salvage procedure in failed total hip replacement** In: Ling RSM, ed. Complications of total hip replacement. London: Churchill Livingstone, 1984:272–281

Haw described the results of excision arthroplasty on 40 hips followed for a mean of 10 years. Patients were satisfied with the operation in unilateral cases as a secondary procedure; it was not satisfactory as a primary operation or when performed bilaterally. Pain relief was satisfactory. One half could walk with no aid or one stick. **Clegg** reviewed 29 patients. Six hips still had a discharging sinus. Complete removal of all cement was essential for healing and lateral guttering was most effective. Pain was relieved but there was much less improvement in function. **Hamblen** discussed the indications and technique. The operation is an effective salvage procedure providing care is taken to removal all bone sequestra and cement fragments. Revision arthroplasty may be considered as a second stage.

Arthrodesis

Watson-Jones, Sir R, Robinson WC **Arthrodesis of the osteoarthritic hip joint** J Bone Joint Surg [Br] 1956;38B:353–377

Callaghan JJ, Brand RA, Pedersen DR **Hip arthrodesis – a long-term follow-up** J Bone Joint Surg [Am] 1985;67A:1328–1335

The authors are conscious that this book is not concerned with operative technique and that arthrodesis of the hip is now rarely indicated. Nevertheless, two articles are considered necessary to indicate basic knowledge on the functional results of this procedure. **Watson-Jones** in 1956 described the the indications and technique, based on a study of 120 patients re-examined 5–20 years after operation. Half of the patients retained normal movement at the knee. There was no back pain in 64%. Photographs are included illustrating function together with ability to sit. This quality of results was only obtained with sound fixation in neutral rotation, no abduction and mild flexion. **Callaghan** has recently described the long-term follow-up of 28 patients who had an arthrodesis 17–50 years previously. Sixty per cent had pain in the ipsilateral knee. There was joint laxity in the ipsilateral knee in a high percentage. These problems were more likely when the hip was fused in abduction. Six patients had undergone total hip arthroplasty for pain in the knee or the back, and in 2 patients a total knee arthroplasty had been performed for pain in the ipsilateral knee.

The Femur

Congenital Femoral Deficiency

Clinical Reviews

Panting AL, Williams PF **Proximal femoral focal deficiency** J Bone Joint Surg [Br] 1978;60B:46–52

Gillespie R, Torode IP **Classification and management of congenital abnormalities of the femur** J Bone Joint Surg [Br] 1983;65B:557–568

Torode IP, Gillespie R **Rotationplasty of the lower limb for congenital defects of the femur** J Bone Joint Surg [Br] 1983;65B:569–573

Fixsen JA **Rotationplasty** J Bone Joint Surg [Br] 1983;65B:529–530

Review Article

Torode IP **Congenital abnormalities of the femur** In: Bennet GC, ed. Paediatric hip disorders. Oxford: Blackwell Scientific Publications, 1987:27–63

Book Reference

Kalamchi A **Congenital lower limb deficiencies.** New York: Springer-Verlag, 1989

Panting discussed and illustrated a classification initially proposed by Amstutz in 1969. Treatment was discussed based on a study of 23 cases. Milder forms are amenable to subtrochanteric osteotomy to correct varus. With progressive deformity, exploration and grafting of the pseudarthrosis is indicated. The management of leg-length inequality is debated. Sixty-nine patients were reviewed by **Gillespie**. Two groups were defined: group I where the hip and knee could be made functional and where sometimes leg equalisation was possible; in group II the hip joint was never normal and the knee joint always useless. A protocol of treatment is suggested. **Torode** discussed the operative technique for combined fusion of the knee and rotationplasty of the limb and its use in 5 patients. In an editorial in the same journal, **Fixsen** debated the value of the "Van Ness procedure" and marshalled the evidence which questioned the value of this operation. **Torode** provided a comprehensive illustrated review of the many problems which this rare condition may present. **Kalamchi** has recently published a small monograph with many illustrations on congenital lower limb deficiencies. Attention is especially drawn to chapters on the development of the lower limb (**Ogden 1–45**), developmental coxa vara (**Schmidt 65–88**), the congenital short femur (**Eilert 89–107**) and proximal femoral focal deficiency (**Krajbich 108–127**). There are also useful sections on treatment, including various amputations and prosthetic management.

The Knee

Anterior Knee Pain

Goodfellow J, Hungerford DS, Woods C **Patellofemoral joint mechanics and pathology 2. Chondromalacia patellae** J Bone Joint Surg [Br] 1976;58B: 291–299

Insall J **Current concepts review: patellar pain** J Bone Joint Surg [Am] 1982; 64A:147–152

Sandow MJ, Goodfellow JW **The natural history of anterior knee pain in adolescents** J Bone Joint Surg [Br] 1985;67B:36–38

Ogilvie-Harris DJ, Jackson RW **The arthroscopic treatment of chondro-malacia patellae** J Bone Joint Surg [Br] 1984;66B:660–665

Fulkerson JP, Shea KP **Current concepts review: disorders of patellofemoral alignment** J Bone Joint Surg [Am] 1990;72A:1424–1429

Goodfellow distinguished between chondromalacia associated with ageing, where there is degeneration on the medial facet, and basal degeneration which is pathological and symptomatic. Surface degeneration was not responsible for patellofemoral pain in young people. Basal degeneration, with fasciculation, may be a cause of intractable patellofemoral pain. The continuing controversies concerning eight recognised causes of patellar pain were reviewed by **Insall**. These included chondromalacia, osteoarthritis, trauma, osteochondritis, the malalignment syndromes, overuse, and sympathetic dystrophy. Principles of treatment were outlined. The place of lateral release, proximal and distal realignment and patella shaving were discussed. Replacement of the patella was indicated for patients with patellofemoral arthritis; a satisfactory outcome can be expected in about half of the patients. **Sandow** studied a group of 54 adolescent girls with anterior knee pain followed for 2–8 years. In many, the symptoms declined with time. It was suggested that surgical treatment seldom need be considered. The arthroscopic treatment of 319 patients with chondromalacia patellae and persistent patellofemoral pain was described by **Ogilvie-Harris**. The aetiology of the pain was divided into four groups: maltracking patella, unstable patella, post-traumatic chondromalacia and idiopathic chondromalacia. Lavage produced early remission in all groups. Although the reasons for success are controversial, arthroscopic surgery has a useful role to play in the management of chondromalacia patellae. The review by **Fulkerson** reflects the interest and advances in knowledge of malalignment of the patella. Accurate radiographic studies, including MRI, may be necessary to identify specific abnormalities. Arthroscopy is valuable when a patient needs operative treatment. Three patterns of malalignment are discussed – tilt, subluxation and a third group with both tilt and subluxation. Crepitus and recurrent effusion suggest degeneration of articular cartilage. The indications for appropriate operative treatment are debated.

Biomechanics

Maquet PGJ **Biomechanics of the knee with application to the pathogenesis and the surgical treatment of osteoarthritis**. 2nd edn. Berlin: Springer-Verlag, 1984:139–266

Maquet's book has been included for reference to his pioneer work in this field. Tibial osteotomy remains the method of choice for treating medial osteoarthrosis with a varus knee (pages 165–186), whereas femoral osteotomy is advocated for the treatment of lateral osteoarthritis with a valgus deformity (pages 218–230). Maquet's advocacy of anterior displacement of the tibial tuberosity is also summarised (pages 144–154).

Radiological Investigation

Senghas RE **Editorial: indications for magnetic resonance imaging** J Bone Joint Surg [Am] 1991;73A:1

Fischer SP, Fox JM, Del Pezo W, Friedman MJ, Snyder SJ, Ferkel RD **Accuracy of diagnoses from magnetic resonance imaging of the knee: a multicentre analysis of 1014 patients** J Bone Joint Surg [Am] 1991;73A:2–10

Raunest J, Oberle K, Loehnert J, Hoetzinger H **The clinical value of magnetic resonance imaging in the evaluation of meniscal disorders** J Bone Joint Surg [Am] 1991;73A:11–16

Senghas debated the arguments for and against MRI bearing in mind the formidable expense of this investigation. **Fischer** found the accuracy of diagnosis from imaging was 89% for the medial meniscus, 88% for the lateral meniscus, and 93% for the anterior cruciate ligament. Results varied substantially at different centres; the reasons for these differences were debated. **Raunest** stated that diagnostic sensitivity was 94% for lesions of the medial meniscus but less for the lateral (78%). MRI has advantages; it is non-invasive and painless and accuracy is not impaired by superimposition of osseous structures. The disadvantages are that it is time consuming, expensive, and provides only a moderate diagnostic accuracy for meniscal disorders such as tears and degeneration.

Chronic Instability

Review Articles

Andrews JR, Axe MJ **The classification of knee ligament instability** Orthop Clin North Am 1985;16:69–82

Noyes FR, McGinniss GH, Grood ES **The variable functional disability of the anterior cruciate ligament-deficient knee** Orthop Clin North Am 1985;16: 47–67

Bollen SR **Trauma: the anterior cruciate ligament. II. Treatment of ACL Rupture** Curr Orthop 1990;4:116–120

Andrews defined the Hughston classification of knee ligament instability. Illustrations are included to describe and demonstrate the lateral and rotatory instabilities. **Noyes** described the syndrome of the anterior cruciate ligament-deficient knee and defined goals of treatment. A functional rating system was produced which gave guidelines for treatment. The possible reconstructive procedures for the chronic ACL-deficient knee are debated. **Bollen** summarised controversies of treatment for patients who present late with symptoms of instability, or fail a course of conservative treatment. The difficulty of assessment of results and therefore comparison of different methods of treatment was stressed.

Clinical Studies

Satku K, Kumar VP, Ngoi SS **Anterior cruciate ligament injuries: to counsel or to operate?** J Bone Joint Surg [Br] 1986;68B:458–461

Frank C, Jackson RW **Lateral substitution for chronic isolated anterior cruciate ligament deficiency** J Bone Joint Surg [Br] 1988;70B:407–411

Bray RC, Flanagan JP, Dandy DJ **Reconstruction for chronic anterior cruciate instability: a comparison of two methods after 6 years** J Bone Joint Surg [Br] 1988;70B:100–105

Fujikawa K, Izeki F, Seedhom BB **Arthroscopy after anterior cruciate reconstruction with the Leeds–Keio ligament** J Bone Joint Surg [Br] 1989; 71B:566–570

Satku studied untreated anterior cruciate ligament injuries reviewed after a mean interval of 6 years; most were able to return to their pre-injury sport, but then deteriorated so that they could not cope. Patients with significant instability during the activities of daily life should be offered operative stabilisation. **Frank** studied 35 patients who had a lateral extra-articular reconstruction alone, followed 5 years after operation; 77% were improved subjectively but only a few patients had "normal knees" and many continued to have minor symptoms of instability with some restriction of activity. The operation failed to return the majority of patients to normality. **Bray** discussed the results of an extra-articular McIntosh procedure. Only 44% had a satisfactory result at 5 years follow-up. The results were not significantly improved by the addition of a carbon fibre replacement for the ACL. **Fujikawa** observed the healing of anterior cruciate ligaments reconstructed with the Leeds–Keio artificial ligament by arthroscopy and, in some, by biopsy. The implant was covered with immature new tissue and a dense vascular network crossed its surface; the new ligament did have the arthroscopic appearance of a normal ACL. A scaffold type of artificial ligament may be effective, but long-term results are not known.

Book Reference

Allen WC, Henstorf JE **Knee ligament reconstruction** In: Evarts CM, ed. Surgery of the musculoskeletal system. 2nd edn, Vol 4. New York: Churchill Livingstone, 1990:3283–3347

Allen supplied a recent comprehensive chapter on this large and changing subject.

Osteochondritis Dissecans

Clinical Studies

Linden B **Osteochondritis dissecans of the femoral condyles: a long-term follow-up study** J Bone Joint Surg [Am] 1977;59A:769–776

Clanton TO, DeLee JC **Osteochondritis dissecans: history, pathophysiology and current treatment concepts** Clin Orthop 1982;167:50–64

Guhl JF **Arthroscopic treatment of osteochondritis dissecans** Clin Orthop 1982;167:65–74

Bradley J, Dandy DJ **Osteochondritis dissecans and other lesions of the femoral condyles** J Bone Joint Surg [Br] 1989;71B:518–522

Bradley J, Dandy DJ **Results of drilling osteochondritis dissecans before skeletal maturity** J Bone Joint Surg [Br] 1989;71B:642–644

Desai SS, Patel MR, Michelli LJ, Silver JW, Lidge RT **Osteochondritis dissecans of the patella** J Bone Joint Surg [Br] 1987;69B:320–325

Linden studied 76 knee joints followed for 30 years. Osteochondritis dissecans in childhood is seldom complicated by secondary gonarthrosis in adult life, regardless of treatment. In contrast, osteochondritis dissecans in the adult is followed by an increasing incidence of gonarthrosis with age, although the symptoms may not develop for 20 years. **Clanton** reviewed the aetiology and treatment. The cause is generally assumed to be multifactorial and related to minor trauma. Conservative treatment is emphasised in the young patient. Drilling is recommended for a loose, unseparated fragment. **Guhl** discussed arthroscopic treatment, based on experience with 50 patients. Ninety per cent healed in a period of 5 months. **Bradley** described the different lesions of the femoral condyle seen in arthroscopy. An attempt was made to define osteochondritis dissecans and separate it from other conditions. The characteristic feature was an expanding concentric lesion at the "classic site" on the medial femoral condyle developing during the 2nd decade of life and progressing to a concave defect in the mature skeleton. **Bradley** later reported the results of arthroscopic drilling of classic lesions in 11 knees with at least 6 months' history and no sign of clinical or radiological improvement. Radiological healing usually occurred. **Desai** reviewed 13 cases of osteochondritis dissecans of the patella followed for some years. This rare condition is the result of repeated minor injuries to the articular surface. Operation is indicated for persistent pain or intra-articular loose bodies. Excision of the fragment and curettage of the crater is recommended.

Osteoarthritis

Upper Tibial Osteomy

1. The Classic

Jackson JP, Waugh W **The technique and complications of upper tibial osteotomy: a review of 226 operations** J Bone Joint Surg [Br] 1974;56B: 236–245

2. Clinical Reviews

Coventry MB **Current concepts review: upper tibial osteotomy for osteoarthritis** J Bone Joint Surg [Am] 1985;67A:1136–1140

Morrey BF **Upper tibial osteotomy for secondary osteoarthritis of the knee** J Bone Joint Surg [Br] 1989;71B:554–559

3. Long-term Follow-up

Vainionpaa S, Laike E, Kirves P, Tiusanen P **Tibial osteotomy for osteoarthritis of the knee: a 5–10 year follow-up study** J Bone Joint Surg [Am] 1981;63A:938–946

Hernigou PH, Medevielle D, Debeyre J, Goutallier D **Proximal tibial osteotomy for osteoarthritis with varus deformity: a 10–13 year follow-up study** J Bone Joint Surg [Am] 1987;69A:332–354

Jackson studied a series of 226 upper tibial osteotomies, with special reference to the complications which occurred with different operative techniques. A wedge osteotomy above the tuberosity was the safest operation. **Coventry** considered osteotomy to be the operation of choice for the relatively young patient with unicompartmental osteoarthritis. **Morrey** discussed the use of proximal tibial osteotomy for secondary degenerative arthritis in 34 patients under 40 years of age. Results were acceptable and preferable to joint replacement. **Vainionpaa** observed 103 knees followed for an average of 7 years. In 83% the result was classified as good or fair. There was, however, a higher incidence of deterioration at 3 years than in previously published series. A total arthroplasty was subsequently necessary in 16 of the 103 knees. **Hernigou** discussed the results of 93 knees that had been treated by proximal tibial opening-wedge osteotomy for varus deformity with osteoarthritis, and followed for 11 years. After 10 years, only 45% had an excellent or good result. However, at 5 years, 90% had a good result. Deterioration occurred at an average of 7 years after osteotomy and was associated with recurrence of pain. Although results deteriorated with time, alignment was a factor in determining long-term results. The best results were obtained in the 20 knees with slight valgus. In these, progression of the arthrosis did not occur. Precise operative technique is therefore essential.

Unicompartmental Replacement

Broughton NS, Newman JH, Baily RAJ **Unicompartmental replacement and high tibial osteotomy for osteoarthritis of the knee – a comparative study after 10–15 years follow-up** J Bone Joint Surg [Br] 1986;68B:447–452

MacKinnon J, Young S, Baily RAJ **The St George sledge for unicompartmental replacement of the knee: a prospective study of 115 cases** J Bone Joint Surg [Br] 1988;70B:217–223

Goodfellow JW, Kershaw CJ, Benson MKD'A, O'Connor JJ **The Oxford knee for unicompartmental osteoarthritis: the first 103 cases** J Bone Joint Surg [Br] 1988;70B:692–701

Kozinn SC, Scott R **Current concepts review: unicondylar knee arthroplasty** J Bone Joint Surg [Am] 1989;71A:145–150

Marmor L **Unicompartmental knee arthroplasty: 10–13 year follow-up study** Clin Orthop 1988;226:14–20

Broughton debated the controversy between the merits of unicompartmental replacement and high tibial osteotomy. A retrospective comparison was made between two groups of patients assessed 5–10 years after operation. The results of unicompartmental replacement were significantly better and this group showed no sign of deterioration. Replacement should be considered, especially in the elderly patient. A prospective study by **McKinnon** of 115 cases followed for 5 years showed 86% excellent or good results. The operation was recommended for osteoarthritis affecting a single tibiofemoral compartment. **Goodfellow** presented experience with the Oxford knee, a resurfacing prosthesis with a meniscal bearing. Pain was relieved in 96%. Absence of the anterior cruciate ligament was associated with a greater incidence of failure and is now considered a contraindication. Osteotomy is recommended for younger patients and unicompartmental arthroplasty for those over 65 years. **Kozinn** discussed patient selection, details of technique and causes of failure. The most appropriate candidate for the operation is more than 60 years old, not obese, not extremely active and has only a mild angular deformity. There must be a good range of motion and minimal flexion contracture. **Marmor** studied 60 knees followed for a minimum of 10 years. Seventy per cent of the patients had satisfactory results. It was important to preserve as much bone stock as possible, and total joint replacement should not be considered on the grounds that the uninvolved compartment may develop arthritis in the future.

Total Knee Arthroplasty

1. Historical

Waugh W **Editorial: knee replacement 1978** J Bone Joint Surg [Br] 1978;60B: 301–303

The rate of change in the development of knee replacement during the last decade has been remarkable. An editorial by **Waugh** depicted the current thought in 1978. A simple solution initially appeared to be a hinge replacement, but there are theoretical and practical arguments against the constraint imposed. Most of the hinged prostheses described in the special number of the 1978 JBJS [Br] have been discarded. Of those discussed, only the Stanmore is still used.

2. Clinical Reviews

Knutson K, Lindstrum A, Lidgren L **Survival of knee arthroplasties: a nation-wide multicentre investigation of 8000 cases** J Bone Joint Surg [Br] 1986;68B: 795–803

Aglietti P, Buzzi R **Posteriorly stabilised total condylar knee replacement: 3–8 years follow-up of 85 knees** J Bone Joint Surg [Br] 1988;70B:211–216

Rorabeck CH, Bourne RB, Nott L **The cemented Kinematic-II and the non-cemented porous-coated anatomic prostheses for total knee replacement: a prospective evaluation** J Bone Joint Surg [Am] 1988;70A:483–490

Insall JN, Binazzi R, Soudry M, Mestriner LA **Total knee arthroplasty** Clin Orthop 1985;192:13–22

Hungerford DS, Krackow KA **Total joint arthroplasty of the knee** Clin Orthop 1985;192:23–33

The results of a prospective nationwide study of knee arthroplasty in 8000 patients were published by **Knutson** in 1986. In osteoarthritis, the probability of the prosthesis remaining after 6 years ranged from 65% for the hinged to 90% for the unicompartmental type. Three compartment prostheses produced intermediate results with 87% survival. The main reason for failure was loosening. **Aglietti** described the use of a posteriorly stabilised total condylar replacement in 85 knees. Excellent or good results were obtained in 90% at 5 years. Replacement of the function of the posterior cruciate ligament does not adversely affect the results at 8 years. Patellofemoral problems provided the most frequent complication, with a 20% incidence of impingement. **Rorabeck** reviewed the improvement of results with the introduction of total condylar prostheses, and especially with metal backing to the tibial component. He compared the results in a prospective non-randomised clinical review with a cemented Kinematic-II prosthesis and a non-cemented porous-coated prosthesis. The follow-up was short but the results of the cemented prosthesis were superior. Current controversies were debated in 1985. **Insall** considered patella resurfacing should be performed in most cases. The debate on cruciate substitution or preservation was unresolved. Correction of deformity was carried out by soft-tissue release and ligament balancing rather than by bone resection. Most failures could be attributed to incorrect ligament balance or incorrect alignment. Cement fixation has proved effective and is preferred. **Hungerford**, however, considered that the majority of total knee components could be fixed rigidly without the addition of cement. They did not tend to deteriorate with time.

3. After Tibial Osteotomy

Staeheli JW, Cass JR, Morrey BF **Condylar total knee arthroplasty after failed proximal tibial osteotomy** J Bone Joint Surg [Am] 1987;69A:28–31

4. After Unicondylar Knee Arthroplasty

Barrett WP, Scott RD **Revision of failed unicondylar unicompartmental knee arthroplasty** J Bone Joint Surg [Am] 1987;69A:1328–1335

The results of condylar knee arthroplasty following a failed tibial osteotomy were studied by **Staeheli**; the results were described in 35 patients observed for 4 years. Eighty-nine per cent were classified as excellent or good. The results were found to be comparable with those after arthroplasty without an osteotomy. No untoward technical difficulties were encountered. Twenty-nine patients who had a revision of a failed knee arthroplasty were studied by **Barrett**. The causes of the failure were discussed, the most common being loosening of one or both components. Technical errors were described. Sixty-six per cent of the failures could be accounted for by preventable errors in selection or surgical technique. At the time of revision, about half of these patients required additional procedures such as bone grafts and the use of special components to carry out posterior cruciate-sparing total knee replacement. There were some failures of revision and the results must be considered inferior to the results of primary total knee arthroplasty.

5. After Tuberculosis of the Knee

Eskola A, Santavirta S, Konttinen YT, Tallroth K, Lindholm ST **Arthroplasty for old tuberculosis of the knee** J Bone Joint Surg [Br] 1988;70B:767–769

Eskola reviewed experience with 6 patients with old tuberculosis of the knee treated by total replacement an average of 35 years after the primary infection. All the patients were markedly improved. Old tuberculosis of the knee can be treated successfully with arthroplasty, but there is a risk of reactivation of disease, and prophylactic drugs are recommended.

6. Problems of the Patella

Merkow RL, Soudry M, Insall JN **Patella dislocation following total knee replacement** J Bone Joint Surg [Am] 1985;67A:1321–1327

Ranawat CS **The patellofemoral joint in total condylar knee arthroplasty: pros and cons based on 5–10 year follow-up observations** Clin Orthop 1986; 205:93–99

Brick GW, Scott RD **The patellofemoral component of total knee arthroplasty** Clin Orthop 1988;231:163–178

In view of their importance, three papers have been included which discuss complications related to the patella. Patellar dislocation is infrequent but can be disabling. **Merkow** described 12 cases. The cause of the dislocation was variable but included incorrect tracking and malrotation of the tibial component. Treatment was by realignment of the quadriceps, and where necessary, component revision. **Ranawat** discussed replacement of the patellofemoral joint. The present trend in the osteoarthritic patella is towards resurfacing. **Brick** illustrated designs and shapes available. The incidence of complications should be reduced by adequate attention at operation to patella tracking and component position.

7. Infection

Johnson DP, Bannister GC **The outcome of infected arthroplasty of the knee** J Bone Joint Surg [Br] 1986;68B:289–291

Grogan TJ, Dorey F, Rollins J, Amstutz HC **Deep sepsis following total knee arthroplasty: 10-year experience at the University of California at Los Angeles Medical Center** J Bone Joint Surg [Am] 1986;68A:226–234

Freeman MAR, Sudlow RA, Casewell MW, Radcliff SS **The management of infected total knee replacements** J Bone Joint Surg [Br] 1985;67B:764–768

Wade PJF, Denham RA **Arthrodesis of the knee after failed knee replacement** J Bone Joint Surg [Br] 1984;66B:362–366

Wilde AH, Stearns KL **Intramedullary fixation for arthrodesis of the knee after infected total knee arthroplasty** Clin Orthop 1989;248:87–92

Johnson described a retrospective analysis of a series of 471 arthroplasties. There were 23 cases of superficial and 25 of deep infection. Superficial infection was minor, but deep infection was predisposed by rheumatoid arthritis, the use of hinged prostheses and superficial infection. Excision of a sinus track, wound debridement and exchange arthroplasty were universally unsuccessful. Arthrodesis was necessary and provided a pain-free gait in 11 out of 12. **Grogan** narrated the course and treatment of 14 infections in 821 knee arthroplasties. Six were haematogenous. The importance of a high index of suspicion and early aggressive treatment was stressed. Salvage may be possible if sepsis is detected early. Nevertheless, only four prostheses were salvaged. **Freeman** discussed the attempt to treat loose infected total knee replacements by a one-stage exchange arthroplasty in 8 patients. The surgical and antibiotic management and results were debated. Arthrodesis of the knee was sometimes required, but fusion can be difficult to obtain. **Wade** described a method of arthrodesis using a simple inexpensive external fixator. Bony union was obtained in all 6 patients. An alternative method of arthrodesis using curved intramedullary rods was discussed by **Wilde**. It was stated to be superior to external fixation in cases of infection, especially with bone loss.

Osteonecrosis

Lotke PA, Ecker ML **Current concepts review: osteonecrosis of the knee** J Bone Joint Surg [Am] 1988;70A:470–473

Aglietti P, Insall JN, Buzzi R, Deschamps G **Idiopathic osteonecrosis of the knee: aetiology, prognosis and treatment** J Bone Joint Surg [Br] 1983; 65B:588–597

Koshino T **The treatment of spontaneous osteonecrosis of the knee by high tibial osteotomy with and without bone grafting or drilling of the lesion** J Bone Joint Surg [Am] 1982;64A:47–58

Bayne O, Langer F, Pritzker KPH, Houpt J, Gross AE **Osteochondral allografts in the treatment of osteonecrosis of the knee** Orthop Clin North Am 1985;16:727–740

Lotke provided a recent review of idiopathic necrosis of the knee which was first reported in 1968. It can occur in either femoral condyle as well as the tibial plateau. The typical patient is elderly and reports sudden onset of pain on the medial side of the knee. The bone scan shows focal increase in activity. The aetiology remains unknown. To date, none of the proposed treatments have been shown to alter the natural history of the early lesion. **Aglietti** described a prospective study of 105 knees with idiopathic necrosis of the femoral condyles. The prognosis is unfavourable with large lesions. Conservative management is advised for small lesions. For large lesions with persistent symptoms, either a high tibial osteotomy or a total knee replacement is advised. Advanced age and a low level of activity favour replacement. **Koshino** obtained good results from high tibial osteotomy, especially when the varus deformity is corrected. Bone grafting or drilling may promote healing of osteonecrosis. Surgical treatment is best performed early. **Bayne** debated the value of osteochondral allografts for this condition, based on the results of 28 operations.

Rheumatoid Arthritis

Review Articles

Beddow FH **Surgical management of the rheumatoid knee** In: Beddow FH, ed. Surgical management of rheumatoid arthritis. London: Wright, 1988: 143–164

Abernethy PJ **Surgery for rheumatoid arthritis 2: Lower limb (ii) Surgery of knee** Curr Orthop 1989;3:3:150–156

Synovectomy

Graham J, Checkets RG **Synovectomy of the knee in rheumatoid arthritis: a long-term follow-up** J Bone Joint Surg [Br] 1973;55B:786–795

Brattstrom H, Czurda R, Gschwend N, Hagena F-W, Kinell I, Kohler G, Mori M, Pavlov VP, Thabe H **Long-term results of knee synovectomy in early cases of rheumatoid arthritis** Clin Rheumatol 1985;4:19–22

Rombouts JJ **Editorial: synovectomy in rheumatoid arthritis** Clin Rheumatol 1985;4:17–18

Sledge CB, Zuckerman JD, Shortkroff S, Zalutsky MR, Venkatesan P, Snyder MA, Barrett WP **Synovectomy of the rheumatoid knee using intra-articular injection of dysprosium-165-ferric hydroxide macroaggregates** J Bone Joint Surg [Am] 1987;69A:970–975

The value of surgical synovectomy of the knee is controversial. **Graham** described the results of synovectomy in 85 patients with rheumatoid arthritis. At review, a minimum of 5 years after surgery, 55% still had improvement in pain. Recurrence of symptoms in nearly all cases was related to recurrence of active disease, but was less likely when surgery was carried out within 3 years of onset of the disease. This paper and others led to the conclusion that the results of surgical synovectomy were disappointing. More recently, **Brattstrom** studied the late results of 508 cases of early synovectomy submitted by nine clinics in a retrospective multicentre follow-up. The observation period was at least 10 years. Sixty-five per cent were reported as subjectively and objectively good, but these clinical results were often associated with radiological deterioration. **Rombouts** concluded that surgical synovectomy was a time-gaining procedure which provided relief of pain, but in the large weight-bearing joints may be associated with significant morbidity. **Abernethy** observed that in the last 20 years there has been a dramatic fall in the number of synovectomies performed in Edinburgh, with a commensurate increase in total knee replacement. The operation can be regarded as a holding procedure allowing joint replacement surgery to be deferred. A straight midline incision is recommended, with preservation of the menisci. **Sledge** reviewed the value of various types of medical synovectomy. One hundred and eleven patients were treated with intra-articular dysprosium ferric hydroxide. It was concluded that this was an effective agent for performing radiation synovectomy and was most useful in knees with minimal radiographic changes.

Total Knee Arthroplasty

Sledge CB, Walker PS **Total knee arthroplasty in rheumatoid arthritis** Clin Orthop 1984;182:127–136

Laskin RS **Total condylar knee replacement in patients who have rheumatoid arthritis: a 10-year follow-up study** J Bone Joint Surg [Am] 1990;72A: 529–535

Sledge discussed the special problems of total knee arthroplasty in rheumatoid arthritis. There is often a valgus external rotation deformity requiring release of the popliteus and lateral structures. Cancellous bone may be weak, requiring precautions to spare the bone–prosthesis interface. The incidence of good and excellent results has risen to 92% with improved prosthetic design and surgical technique. **Laskin** studied a 10-year follow-up of 80 knee replacements. When revision, pain or radiographic evidence of loosening were considered an indication of failure, the 10-year cumulative survival was 75%. **Beddow** reviewed the surgical management of the rheumatoid knee, discussing surgical pathology, synovectomy and total knee arthroplasty. There was no agreement on the management of the patella, except that it should not be removed. Deterioration in overall assessment was invariably due to rheumatoid involvement elsewhere. **Abernethy** debated the value of knee arthroplasty based on a series of 275 total condylar replacements. The main indication is severe pain. Stiffness may be unrewarding to treat since recovery of function is unpredictable. Where the patella is resurfaced, there is less anterior knee pain and better function. The patella must track easily in the femoral groove during passive flexion and extension. Specific problems which may arise in the rheumatoid knee are postoperative stiffness, gross malalignment and bony defects.

Reflex Sympathetic Dystrophy

Katz MM, Hungerford DS **Reflex sympathetic dystrophy affecting the knee** J Bone Joint Surg [Br] 1987;69B:797–803

Ogilvie-Harris DJ, Roscoe M **Reflex sympathetic dystrophy of the knee** J Bone Joint Surg [Br] 1987;69B:804–806

Cooper DE, DeLee JC, Ramamurthy S **Reflex sympathetic dystrophy of the knee: treatment using continuous epidural anaesthesia** J Bone Joint Surg [Am] 1989;71A:365–369

Katz reviewed 36 patients with this condition. Diagnostic criteria were strict and included pain, loss of function, vasomotor instability and hypersensitivity. The importance of injuries or operation about the patellofemoral joint were emphasised. Those who underwent sympathetic blockade within 1 year of onset obtained better results than those treated later. Treatment was by sympathetic manipulation, and early diagnosis remains the key to successful management. **Ogilvie-Harris** reported on 19 cases. Skyline radiography and bone scintigraphy are valuable as important diagnostic tools. Treatment included analgesia, sympathetic blockade, manipulation, and continuous passive motion. Despite this regimen, no patient regained a normal knee. **Cooper** described the results of treatment using continuous epidural analgesia, manipulation under anaesthetic and continuous passive motion. Good results were reported in 14 patients. The diagnosis of reflex sympathetic dystrophy must be considered in any patient who has excessive pain for the severity of the injury with atrophic changes in the skin. Some patients had undergone inconclusive arthroscopic surgery.

The Discoid Lateral Meniscus

Smillie IS, **The congenital discoid meniscus** J Bone Joint Surg [Br] 1948; 30B:671–682

Dickhaut SC, DeLee JC **The discoid lateral meniscus syndrome** J Bone Joint Surg [Am] 1982;64A:1068–1073

Smillie described and photographed 29 discoid menisci. Three types were recognised. They were called primitive, infantile and intermediate. **Dickhaut** described a complete type of discoid lateral meniscus that is frequently asymptomatic, while the Wrisberg-ligament type produces the clinical syndrome that is usually associated with discoid lateral meniscus. There is a clinical syndrome of a snapping knee, due to the meniscus being displaced into the intercondylar notch by the attachment to the Wrisberg ligament.

Popliteal Cysts

The Classic

Baker WM **The formation of abnormal synovial cysts in connection with the joints** St Bart's Hosp Rep 1885;21:177–190

Baker drew attention to the formation of synovial cysts as a consequence of disease, especially of osteoarthritis; some were caused by tuberculosis and some by rheumatoid arthritis. Fluctuation may not be present from the cyst to the joint, but its absence does not disprove a connection. Abnormal cysts may also be found in connection with other joints, including the shoulder, elbow, hip and ankle.

Clinical Studies

Myles AB **Posterior synovial leaks in arthritis of the knee** Proc R Soc Med 1971;64:262–264

Pinder IM **Treatment of the popliteal cyst in the rheumatoid knee** J Bone Joint Surg [Br] 1973;55B:119–125

Dinham JM **Popliteal cysts in children: the case against surgery** J Bone Joint Surg [Br] 1975;57B:69–71

The diagnosis and treatment of popliteal cysts is controversial. **Myles** discussed those associated with rheumatoid arthritis. A cyst may leak in various ways and extend inferiorly into the calf; it may produce chronic leg oedema and must be differentiated from a venous thrombosis. **Pinder** debated the possible treatment of popliteal cysts in rheumatoid disease by the reduction of raised intracapsular pressure by anterior synovectomy. **Dinham** reviewed the natural history of 120 popliteal cysts in children. Most disappear spontaneously and operation is usually not necessary.

Meniscal Cysts

Wroblewski BM **Trauma and the cystic meniscus: review of 500 cases** Injury 1973;4:319–321

Flynn M, Kelly JP **Local excision of cyst of lateral meniscus of knee without recurrence** J Bone Joint Surg [Br] 1976;58B:88–89

Barrie HJ **The pathogenesis and significance of meniscal cysts** J Bone Joint Surg [Br] 1979;61B:184–189

Wroblewski analysed 500 cases. Cystic meniscus is a common lesion not confined to the young athletic male or to the lateral meniscus. A cyst with an undamaged meniscus was found in 50%. A parrot-beak tear was the most common single abnormality. **Flynn** discussed excision of the cyst only in patients shown to have no concomitant tear of the cartilage. The rehabilitation period was less, and recurrence of the cyst did not occur. **Barrie** reported a study of 112 surgically excised specimens of cystic menisci, all of which showed horizontal tears. Tracks were often demonstrable, linking the tear to the cyst. It was concluded that the cysts were fuelled by synovial fluid. The accepted concept of a primary "myxoid degeneration" is not correct.

The Tibia

Tibia Vara (Blount's Disease)

The Classic

Langenskiold A, Riska EB **Tibia vara (osteochondrosis deformans tibiae): a survey of 71 cases** J Bone Joint Surg [Am] 1964;46A:1405–1420

Langenskiold reported 61 cases of the infantile type of tibia vara and 10 cases of the adolescent type. Six different stages of the diseases are presented.

Clinical Studies

Smith CF **Current concepts review: tibia vara (Blount's disease)** J Bone Joint Surg [Am] 1982;64A:630–632

Kumar SJ, Pizzutillo PD **Treatment of Blount's disease** In: Uhthoff HK, Wiley JJ, eds. Behaviour of the growth plate. New York: Raven Press, 1987: 299–307

Hofmann A, Jones RE, Herring JA **Blount's disease after skeletal maturity** J Bone Joint Surg [Am] 1982;64A:1004–1009

Smith reviewed this rare condition; it presents as a severe bowing and internal rotation of the tibiae in childhood. The diagnostic radiographic finding is medial metaphyseal fragmentation. Eighty per cent of patients with the infantile type have bilateral deformity. The disease is progressive and the treatment is corrective (tibial and fibular) osteotomy. Adolescent tibia vara is related to trauma with an onset after the age of 8 years. **Kumar** considered night bracing could be tried for children up to 3 years of age. The deformity is complex, and to achieve correction, various types of proximal tibial osteotomy have been proposed. For adolescent tibia vara an oblique proximal tibial osteotomy gives excellent results. **Hofmann** studied 12 patients 12 years after osteotomy. Most were symptomatic, with early degenerative changes. A poor final outcome was related to physeal damage. Early osteotomy must be performed to prevent this damage.

Congenital Pseudarthrosis

Boyd HB **Pathology and natural history of congenital pseudarthrosis of the tibia** Clin Orthop 1982;166:5–13

Morrissy RT, Riseborough EJ, Hall JE **Congenital pseudarthosis of the tibia** J Bone Joint Surg [Br] 1981;63B:367–375

Umber JS, Moss SW, Coleman SS **Surgical treatment of congenital pseudarthrosis of the tibia** Clin Orthop 1982;166:28–33

Pho RWH, Levack B, Satku K, Patradul A **Free vascularised fibular graft in the treatment of congenital pseudarthrosis of the tibia** J Bone Joint Surg [Br] 1985;67B:64–70

Jacobsen ST, Crawford AH, Millar EA, Steele HH **The Syme amputation in patients with congenital pseudarthrosis of the tibia** J Bone Joint Surg [Am] 1983;65A:533–537

Paterson DC **Congenital pseudarthrosis of the tibia: an overview** Clin Orthop 1989;247:44–54

Based upon the pathology and radiology of 14 cases, **Boyd** described six types of congenital pseudarthrosis. The pathology of the most frequent (type II) is an aggressive osteolytic fibromatosis. Failure of treatment is due to a recurrence of the fibromatosis, which can remove living bone or a dead bone graft. **Morrissy** reviewed 40 cases treated in Boston and Toronto. At the time of review, 14 patients had undergone amputation. Congenital pseudarthrosis of the tibia is a biological problem and not merely a mechanical one. The many problems of surgical treatment are described by **Umber**, based on 14 cases from Salt Lake City. Dual tibio-fibular intramedullary rodding with autogenous bone grafting is the treatment of choice. **Pho** described five cases successfully treated by a free vascularised fibula graft. Surgical treatment is described in detail; it includes radical excision of abnormal bone and permits bone lengthening and correction of deformity. **Jacobsen** considered that when an amputation was necessary, a Syme can be recommended. With a simple orthosis, even if the pseudarthrosis remains ununited, the child can engage in normal activities. Experience was described with 8 patients followed for an average of 6 years. **Paterson** has provided an overview of this subject. He had achieved union in 24 of 30 pseudarthroses using intramedullary fixation and cancellous bone grafting, followed by electrical stimulation. Reference is also made to the use of the Ilizarov external fixator in the treatment of this rare condition.

The Ankle

There is still controversy concerning the merits of arthrodesis versus arthroplasty.

Arthrodesis

Ratliff AHC **Compression arthrodesis of the ankle** J Bone Joint Surg [Br] 1959;41B:524–534

Baciu CC **A simple technique for arthrodesis of the ankle** J Bone Joint Surg [Br] 1986;68B:266–267

Lynch AF, Bourne RB, Rorabeck CH **The long-term results of ankle arthrodesis** J Bone Joint Surg [Br] 1988;70B:113–116

Helm R **The results of ankle arthrodesis** J Bone Joint Surg [Br] 1990; 72B: 141–143

In 1959, **Ratliff** reviewed the results of compression arthrodesis of the ankle performed on 55 patients, largely by Mr J. Charnley. Bony fusion occurred in 91%, with a good or excellent subjective result in 88%. The best position for arthrodesis is at, or close to, the right-angle. **Baciu** described a simple rapid operation using a Milling cutter to obtain a cylindrical bone graft, which is introduced having been reversed. Bony fusion occurred in a high percentage, but the technique can only be employed where there is no deformity at the joint. The results of 62 ankle arthrodeses, mostly performed for osteoarthritis, were described by **Lynch**. Compression arthrodesis was associated with the highest incidence of complications and an anterior sliding graft gave the most satisfactory results. Most patients had excellent pain relief and could walk independently with a slight limp. **Helm** presented the results of 47 compression arthrodeses performed for osteoarthritis. Ankle arthrodesis can give very good results in patients with disabling arthritis, but there is a significant risk of complications. Arthrodesis should be reserved for patients in whom severe pain is the main complaint. The importance of avoiding a varus or valgus position of the heel was stressed.

Arthroplasty

Lachiewicz PF, Inglis AE, Ranawat CS **Total ankle replacement in rheumatoid arthritis** J Bone Joint Surg [Am] 1984;66A:340–343

Bolton-Maggs BG, Sudlow RA, Freeman MAR **Total ankle arthroplasty – a long-term review of the London Hospital experience** J Bone Joint Surg [Br] 1985;67B:785–790

Hamblen DL **Editorial: can the ankle joint be replaced?** J Bone Joint Surg [Br] 1985;67B:689–690

Kirkup J **Rheumatoid arthritis and ankle surgery** Ann Rheum Dis 1990; 49:Suppl 2:837–844

Lachiewicz portrayed the difficult problems presented with severe rheumatoid disease. There is often involvement of the subtalar and mid-tarsal joints, and therefore no compensatory movement. Nevertheless, on a short follow-up he had obtained good results with relief of pain using the Mayo type of ankle replacement. **Bolton-Maggs** reported a retrospective study of 62 ankle arthroplasties. There was a high complication rate and poor long-term results. Arthrodesis was therefore recommended as the treatment of choice for the painful, stiff arthritic ankle, regardless of the underlying pathological process. **Hamblen** debated design concept and possible future development. **Kirkup** described the results of 57 arthroplasties and followed for a mean of 4 years. The joint was spherocentric, with a polyethylene tibial component and a steel talar implant. Results were described as modest and resembled those of the earlier versions of knee prostheses. For severely disabled rheumatoid patients with bilateral tarsal ankylosis and crippling ankle pain, joint replacement is justified on one side and sometimes on both. Careful patient selection is essential.

Osteochondritis Dissecans

Bauer M, Jonsson K, Linden B **Osteochondritis dissecans of the ankle: a 20-year follow-up study** J Bone Joint Surg [Br] 1987;69B:93–96

Bauer described observations on 30 patients with osteochondritis dissecans, followed for an average of 21 years. Most patients had only minor radiographic changes and symptoms. Two patients only had developed osteoarthritis.

The Foot

Club Foot

The Classic

Wynne-Davies R **Family studies and the cause of congenital club foot. Talipes equinovarus, talipes calcaneovalgus and metatarsus varus** J Bone Joint Surg [Br] 1964;46B:445–463

Wynne-Davies studied the family history and associated congenital abnormalities, in 635 patients with talipes equinovarus. The overall incidence is approximately 1 in 1000. If one child in a family has the condition, the chance of an affected sibling is 1 in 35.

Aetiology and Pathology

Cowell HR, Wein BK **Current concepts review: genetic aspects of club foot** J Bone Joint Surg [Am] 1980;62A:1381–1384

Main BJ, Crider RJ **An analysis of residual deformity in club feet submitted to early operation** J Bone Joint Surg [Br] 1978;60B:536–543

Swann M, Lloyd-Roberts GC, Catterall A **The anatomy of uncorrected club feet: a study of rotation deformity** J Bone Joint Surg [Br] 1969;51B:263–269

Cowell summarised the environmental and genetic factors which may cause club foot. The condition is usually idiopathic. Contributions to the deformity made by metatarsus primus varus, medial subluxation of the navicular, and angulation of the neck of the talus were debated by **Main**. He considered that medial subluxation of the navicular was the most important and that early relocation at the talonavicular joint correlated with success of treatment. **Swann** discussed the anatomy of the established deformity with particular reference to abnormal torsion.

Treatment

Porter RW **Congenital talipes equinovarus. I. Resolving and resistant deformities** J Bone Joint Surg [Br] 1987;69B:822–825

Porter RW **Congenital talipes equinovarus. II. A staged method of surgical treatment** J Bone Joint Surg [Br] 1987;69B:826–831

Tayton K, Thompson P **Relapsing club feet: late results of delayed operation** J Bone Joint Surg [Br] 1979;61B:474–480

Addison A, Fixsen JA, Lloyd-Roberts GC **A review of the Dillwyn Evans type collateral operation in severe club feet** J Bone Joint Surg [Br] 1983;65B: 12–14

Turco VJ **Resistant congenital club foot – one-stage posteromedial release with internal fixation. A follow-up report of the 15-year experience** J Bone Joint Surg [Am] 1979;61A:805–814

Hutchins PM, Foster BK, Paterson DC, Cole EA **Long-term results of early surgical release in club feet** J Bone Joint Surg [Br] 1985;67B:791–799

McKay DW **New concept of and approach to clubfoot treatment. III. Evaluation and results** J Pediatr Orthop 1983;3:141–148

Simons GW **Complete subtalar release in club feet. II. Comparison with less extensive procedures** J Bone Joint Surg [Am] 1985;67A:1056–65

Porter compared those children whose deformity resolved with conservative treatment and those who required surgical correction. He suggested that there are two distinct populations, those that resolve rapidly and are then indistinguishable from normal, and those that persist. This distinction is of considerable importance, especially in the assessment of the results of treatment. **Porter** described the results of a personal series of 125 feet where a two-stage surgical correction had been performed. Hindfoot correction was carried out at 6 weeks, followed by a second-stage medial forefoot correction. The continuing controversies of surgical treatment such as timing, correction and its maintenance were debated. **Tayton** described in detail the operation of soft-tissue release and calcaneocuboid fusion published by Dillwyn Evans in 1961. A long-term review of 118 club feet was presented, the average age of the patients being 17 years. Early operation had been deliberately delayed by a policy of prolonged conservative treatment. The method was generally successful, but only 37% had full anatomical correction. The paper by **Addison** has been included since the results of treatment by the Dillwyn Evans operation are described in patients who had undergone previous surgery elsewhere. They were probably difficult cases. The results were satisfactory in 30 out of 45 patients. **Turco** reviewed a personal experience with 240 resistant congenital club feet (176 patients) treated surgically by a one-stage posteromedial release with internal fixation. There were 84% excellent or good results; the best results were in children who were operated on between the ages of 1 and 2 years. The results of treatment of 252 club feet by early posterior release were reviewed by **Hutchins** after a follow-up of 16 years. The surgical technique 6–8 weeks after birth was described. A satisfactory result was obtained in 81%. The range of ankle movement was a major factor in determining the functional result and this was influenced by the flattening of the talus. **McKay** designed a one-stage subtalar soft-tissue release to correct the horizontal subtalar rotation of the calcaneus. **Simons** designed a complete subtalar release and considered that this provided a higher percentage of satisfactory results than did the less extensive soft-tissue procedures.

Review Article

Cummings RJ, Lovell WW **Current concepts review: operative treatment of congenital idiopathic club foot** J Bone Joint Surg [Am] 1988;70A:1108–1112

Cummings debated the current controversies (1988). A universally accepted method of classification of the severity of the deformity is lacking. There is no standardised method of evaluating the results. There is still no agreement as to the choice of operative procedures. Initial treatment is by gentle corrective manipulation, and application of serial splinting. Surgical correction at an early age without attempts at non-operative correction should be discouraged. The one-stage posteromedial soft-tissue release procedure described by **Turco** is still favoured by many. The **McKay** procedure is growing in favour. Soft-tissue procedures necessitate meticulous dissection to achieve complete and lasting correction.

Tarsal Coalition

Mitchell GP, Gibson JMC **Excision of the calcaneonavicular bar for painful spasmodic flat foot** J Bone Joint Surg [Br] 1967;49B:281–287

Leonard MA **The inheritance of tarsal coalition and its relationship to spastic flat foot** J Bone Joint Surg [Br] 1974;56B:520–526

Mosier KM, Asher M **Tarsal coalitions and peroneal spastic flat foot: a review** J Bone Joint Surg [Am] 1984;66A:977–984

Mitchell described the results of excision of the calcaneonavicular bar in 28 patients. Excision was a good procedure in the younger patient with painful spasmodic flat foot of recent origin. The indications for the operation and technique were described. **Leonard** studied the inheritance of tarsal coalition. The families of 31 patients were analysed. Thirty-nine per cent were found to have some type of tarsal coalition. **Mosier** reviewed the clinical presentation, radiological appearances and treatment of tarsal coalition. Resection of the talocalcaneal coalition is controversial. Arthrodesis remains the final form of surgical treatment for the relief of symptomatic tarsal coalition, but is seldom necessary.

Congenital Vertical Talus

The Classic

Lloyd-Roberts GC, Spence AJ **Congenital vertical talus** J Bone Joint Surg [Br] 1958;40B:33–41

Clinical Studies

Coleman SS, Stelling FH, Jarrett J **Pathomechanics and treatment of congenital vertical talus** Clin Orthop 1970;70:62–72

Jacobsen ST, Crawford AH **Congenital vertical talus** J Pediatr Orthop 1983; 3:306–310

Hamanishi C **Congenital vertical talus: classification with 69 cases and new measurement system** J Pediatr Orthop 1984;4:318–326

The clinical and radiological features of 32 feet with congenital vertical talus were described by **Lloyd-Roberts**. The differential diagnosis of this condition from flat foot, talipes calcaneus and uncorrected club foot was discussed. **Coleman** discussed the complicated pathology of this rare condition. Two major types exist, type I in which the calcaneocuboid relationship is normal, and type II which is associated with a calcaneocuboid dislocation or subluxation. An operative technique for treatment is illustrated. **Jacobsen** discussed experience with the Coleman two-stage realignment procedure in 17 feet. Forty-four cases of idiopathic vertical talus were reviewed by **Hamanishi**. He classified the cases into five groups and introduced methods which assessed the obliquity of the talus, and thus influenced management. Children who could be treated by serial casts and open reduction obtained the best results. Triple arthrodesis may be necessary in a child of 12 years or older.

Rupture of the Tibialis Posterior Tendon

Mann RA, Thompson FM **Rupture of the posterior tibial tendon causing flat foot: surgical treatment** J Bone Joint Surg [Am] 1985;67A:556–561

Rupture of the posterior tibial tendon results in a progressive, painful flat-foot deformity. **Mann** provided a useful reference to this condition; 17 patients are reported who were surgically treated with a transfer of the flexor digitorum longus tendon into the navicular, or an advancement of the posterior tibial tendon. Twelve patients had an excellent result which did not deteriorate with time.

Pes Cavus

Jahss MH **Tarsometatarsal truncated-wedge arthrodesis for pes cavus and equinovarus deformity of the fore part of the foot** J Bone Joint Surg [Am] 1980;62A:713–722

Bradley GW, Coleman SS **Treatment of the calcaneocavus foot deformity** J Bone Joint Surg [Am] 1981;63A:1159–1166

The indications, contraindications and technique of truncated wedge arthrodesis for various types of pes cavus were discussed by **Jahss**, including the complications. The results were considered excellent in 34 patients. **Bradley** discussed the calcaneocavus foot, based on a study of 19 cases. The deformity is progressive, disabling, and results from paralysis of the gastrocnemius and soleus muscles. Treatment is always surgical and demands aggressive correction of the deformity and restoration of muscle balance.

Hallux Valgus – The Adult

The Classic

Bonney G, Macnab I **Hallux valgus and hallux rigidus: a critical survey of operative results** J Bone Joint Surg [Br] 1952;34B:366–385

Clinical Studies

Fitzgerald JAW **A review of the long-term results of arthrodesis of the first metatarsophalangeal joint** J Bone Joint Surg [Br] 1969;51B:488–493

Henry APJ, Waugh W **The use of foot prints in assessing the results of operations for hallux valgus: a comparison of Keller's operation and arthrodesis** J Bone Joint Surg [Br] 1975;57B:478–481

Turnbull T, Grange W **A comparison of Keller's arthroplasty and distal metatarsal osteotomy in the treatment of adult hallux valgus** J Bone Joint Surg [Br] 1986;68B:132–137

Coughlin MJ, Mann RA **Arthrodesis of the first metatarsophalangeal joint as salvage for the failed Keller procedure** J Bone Joint Surg [Am] 1987;69A: 68–75

O'Doherty DP, Lowrie IG, Magnussen PA, Gregg PJ **The management of the painful first metatarsophalangeal joint in the older patient: arthrodesis or Keller's arthroplasty?** J Bone Joint Surg [Br] 1990;72B:839–842

Bonney in 1952 surveyed the results of 518 operations for hallux valgus and rigidus. He considered there was nothing to choose between the results of the Keller and Mayo operations. In general, results of arthroplasty in the adult for hallux valgus were "reasonable", but nevertheless some results were disappointing. **Fitzgerald** reviewed 100 cases of arthrodesis of the first metatarsophalangeal joint after a postoperative interval of at least 10 years. Seventy-seven per cent were completely satisfied; only 9% were dissatisfied. The major factors leading to poor results were malposition of the arthrodesis and interphalangeal osteoarthritis. The increasing use of pressure studies was described by **Henry**. He compared the results of Keller's operation and arthrodesis in a review of 170 feet. Patterns of weight bearing were compared; after arthrodesis the big toe bore weight in 80% compared with 40% after a Keller's operation. Ability to bear weight on the big toe is related to the incidence of metatarsalgia. **Turnbull** described a prospective trial which compared the results of distal osteotomy with a Keller's arthroplasty in 33 patients over the age of 30 years. The series is small and the follow-up short. The range of movement at the metatarsophalangeal joint was better maintained after osteotomy and degenerative changes did not compromise a successful result. The paper by

Coughlin has been included as a reminder that poor results may follow a Keller's procedure, and that there appears to be no comprehensive recent long-term study on the results of that operation. **O'Doherty** reported the results of a prospective randomised trial comparing Keller's arthroplasty and arthrodesis of the first metatarsophalangeal joint for symptomatic hallux valgus and hallux rigidus in the older patient. In 81 patients with a minimum of 2 years follow-up, both procedures gave a similar degree of patient satisfaction. As there were no advantages to arthrodesis and since a small number of arthrodesed toes required revision, Keller's arthroplasty was considered to be the better operation. The authors were also unable to trace a study of the long-term value of silastic implants in the metatarsophalangeal joint of the great toe.

Hallux Valgus – The Young Adult

The Classic

Mitchell CL, Fleming JL, Allan R, Glenney C, Sanford GA **Osteotomy bunionectomy for hallux valgus** J Bone Joint Surg [Am] 1958;40A:41–60

Clinical Studies

Piggott H **The natural history of hallux valgus in adolescence and early adult life** J Bone Joint Surg [Br] 1960;42B:749–760

Helal B **Surgery for adolescent hallux valgus** Clin Orthop 1981;157:50–63

Grace D, Hughes J, Klenerman L **A comparison of Wilson and Hohmann osteotomies in the treatment of hallux valgus** J Bone Joint Surg [Br] 1988; 70B:236–241

Horne G, Tancer T, Ford N **Chevron osteotomy for treatment of hallux valgus** Clin Orthop 1984;183:32–36

In 1958, **Mitchell** described his experience with over 400 operations performed for hallux valgus with metatarsus primus varus. The precise technique of this osteotomy is illustrated, and the cause of technical failures discussed. Although the original technique has been modified by some surgeons, this operation is still widely used. **Piggott** discussed the different ways in which increased valgus of the great toe may occur. A distinction was made between three types: the congruous, the deviated and the subluxated. Once subluxation has occurred, progression of the deformity is likely. **Helal** provided a critical review with diagrams of the large number of operations described for adolescent hallux valgus. The paper by **Grace** has been included since it compared results of the Wilson and Hohmann osteotomies. There were no poor results and no differences between the two operations in patient satisfaction, pain relief, appearance, footwear and walking ability. **Horne** described the technique and results of a Chevron osteotomy in 51 patients observed for 3 years. Increased mechanical stability is considered to permit a shorter period of postoperative immobilisation.

Hallux Rigidus

McMaster MJ **The pathogenesis of hallux rigidus** J Bone Joint Surg [Br] 1978;60B:82–87

Citron N, Neil M **Dorsal wedge osteotomy of the phalanx for hallux rigidus – long-term results** J Bone Joint Surg [Br] 1987;69B:835–837

Fitzgerald JAW **A review of the long-term results of arthrodesis of the first metatarsophalageal joint** J Bone Joint Surg [Br] 1969;51B:488–493

McMaster studied the pathological features of hallux rigidus. Characteristic osteochondral lesions occur on the metatarsal head and account for the limitation of dorsiflexion at the joint. **Citron** observed the results of a dorsal wedge osteotomy of the proximal phalanx in 8 patients followed for an average of 22 years. This procedure affords good results in the adolescent female. **Fitzgerald** considered arthrodesis to be the operation of choice for hallux rigidus, with a high percentage of satisfactory results. The ideal position for fusion was between 20° and 40° of dorsiflexion, 20° and 30° of valgus, and neutral rotation.

The Rheumatoid Hindfoot

Heywood AWB **Supramalleolar osteotomy in the management of the rheumatoid hindfoot** Clin Orthop 1983;177:76–81

Stockley I, Betts RP, Rowley DI, Getty CJM, Duckworth T **The importance of the valgus hindfoot in forefoot surgery in rheumatoid arthritis** J Bone Joint Surg [Br] 1990;72B:705–708

Kitaoka HB **Rheumatoid hindfoot** Orthop Clin North Am 1989;20:4:593–604

Heywood stressed that, although hindfoot involvement is common in rheumatoid arthritis, indications for surgery are rare. Osteotomy may be a useful procedure where there is fixed deformity or unremitting pain. **Stockley** drew attention to the importance of a valgus hindfoot in rheumatoid arthritis and observed that patients with these deformities tend to have high forefoot pressures. **Kitaoka** discussed the variable clinical course without treatment. The initial treatment generally should be non-operative. Shoe modifications may be helpful. For advanced arthrosis, a selective arthrodesis, such as talonavicular, may be appropriate.

The Rheumatoid Forefoot

Fowler AW **A method of forefoot reconstruction** J Bone Joint Surg [Br] 1959;41B:507–513

Kates A, Kessel L, Kay A **Arthroplasty of the forefoot** J Bone Joint Surg [Br] 1967;49B:552–557

Barton NJ **Arthroplasty of the forefoot in rheumatoid arthritis** J Bone Joint Surg [Br] 1973;55B:126–133

Craxford AD, Stevens J, Park C **Management of the deformed rheumatoid forefoot: a comparison of conservative and surgical methods** Clin Orthop 1982;166:121–126

Mann RA, Thompson FM **Athrodesis of the first metatarsophalangeal joint for hallux valgus in rheumatoid arthritis** J Bone Joint Surg [Am] 1984; 66A:687–692

In 1959, **Fowler** described a forefoot resection with removal of the metatarsal heads, the exposure being performed through a dorsal skin incision. An ellipse of skin was also removed from the plantar surface to restore the position of the metatarsal pad. The principles of this procedure have gained wide acceptance. **Kates** modified this operation, resecting the metatarsal heads through the plantar surface of the foot. **Barton** reviewed the results of operations on 65 feet. The subjective results were remarkably good, but the most common cause of persistent pain was prominence of one metatarsal stump. There was no major difference in the results of three different techniques. **Craxford** compared the late results of surgery with conservative treatment with surgical shoes. The study was retrospective; it suggested that surgery relieved pain initially but the recurrence rate of metatarsalgia was high. There was little difference between the outcomes of non-operative and surgical treatment. The results of reconstruction of the forepart of the foot in rheumatoid arthritis by arthrodesis of the first metatarsophalangeal joint were reviewed by **Mann**. He concluded that this procedure provided stability, permitted the wearing of ordinary shoes, and with excision arthroplasty of the other toes, relieved disabling pain.

Morton's Metatarsalgia

Mulder JD **The causative mechanism in Morton's metatarsalgia** J Bone Joint Surg [Br] 1951;33B:94–95

Bossley CJ, Cairney PC **The intermetatarsophalangeal bursa: its significance in Morton's metatarsalgia** J Bone Joint Surg [Br] 1980;62B:184–187

Guiloff RJ, Scadding JW, Klenerman L **Morton's metatarsalgia: clinical, electrophysiological and histological observations** J Bone Joint Surg [Br] 1984; 66B:586–591

In 1951, **Mulder** described a characteristic click when examining patients with a painful forefoot, and noted that at operation a neuroma was adherent to the intermetatarsal bursa. **Bossley** investigated the characteristics of the intermetatarsophalangeal bursa. **Guiloff** investigated 16 patients suffering from Morton's metatarsalgia, and these included nerve conduction studies. There is now general agreement that the pain of Morton's metatarsalgia is due to the observed neural changes, but there is still controversy about the pathogenesis of these changes.

The Diabetic Foot

Newman JH **Spontaneous dislocation in diabetic neuropathy: a report of 6 cases** J Bone Joint Surg [Br] 1979;61B:484–488

Newman JH **Non-infective disease of the diabetic foot** J Bone Joint Surg [Br] 1981;63B:593–596

Duckworth T, Boulton AJM, Betts RP, Flanks CJ, Ward JD **Plantar pressure measurements and the prevention of ulceration in the diabetic foot** J Bone Joint Surg [Br] 1985;67B:79–85

Harrelson JM **Management of the diabetic foot** Orthop Clin North Am 1989; 20:4:605–619

Wagner FW **Infections of the foot in diabetes** In: Chapman MW, ed. Operative orthopaedics 3. Philadelphia: J B Lippincott Co, 1988:1833–1843

Newman (1979) described the clinical details of 6 patients who developed spontaneous dislocation in the foot or ankle, and who suffered from diabetic neuropathy. Later (1981) he described six different types of non-infective bone and joint pathology amongst 67 patients with diabetic neuropathy. These conditions differ from osteomyelitis. A Charcot osteoarthropathy is the most common condition. **Duckworth** described static and dynamic measurements of foot pressure in diabetic patients, with normal subjects as controls. Areas of abnormally high pressure under the foot were outlined. Suitable means were devised to protect the foot and prevent ulceration. **Harrelson** illustrated experience from a clinic specifically designed to provide diabetic foot care. The cause of damage may be divided into three categories: ischaemia, soft-tissue neuropathy and arthropathy. Ischaemia may result from both large- and small-vessel disease. The most common presenting complaint is a painful ulcer of short duration. Amputations may be preferable to continued conservative care. Neuropathic ulceration is the product of decreased sensation and deformity. Pressure relief by conservative or surgical means is required for healing. Neuropathic ulcers require protection from weight bearing and orthotic control. A chapter by **Wagner** is included since it reflects the increased interest of orthopaedic surgeons in this subject. Centres are now reporting superior results when a specialised team assesses and treats the diabetic foot.

Toenail Disorders

Greig JD, Anderson JH, Ireland AJ, Anderson JR **The surgical treatment of ingrowing toenails** J Bone Joint Surg [Br] 1991;73B:131–133

Two prospective studies of ingrowing-toenail management were conducted. Recurrence rates were high following simple avulsion or nail-edge excision, and these methods of treatment should not be practised. Nail-edge excision with phenolisation is a logical and effective treatment where conservative management has failed, and for recurrence following a surgical procedure.

Author Index

Subject Index

Hypochondroplasia 46

Ibuprofen in ankylosing spondylitis 33
Idiopathic chronic adhesive capsulitis 62
Iliopsoas transplantation 25
Impingement lesions 57
Incomplete anterior interosseous nerve
    syndrome 54
Indomethacin in ankylosing spondylitis 33
Infantile malignant osteopetrosis 20
Infection 2–7
    bone and joint 44
    hip replacement 141, 144–5
    in sickle-cell disease 44
    joint replacement 143–5
    knee arthroplasty 162–3
    osteomyelitis 2–5
    suppurative arthritis in the child 5–6
    tuberculosis of bone and joint 6–7
Intermetatarsophalangeal bursa 181
Interphalangeal joint, silicone implants 73
Intertrochanteric osteotomy 129
Intervertebral disc space infection 4
Intramedullary haemorrhage in avascular
    necrosis 42

Joint replacement
    infection 143–5
    sarcoma in 11
Juvenile chronic arthritis 139

Kienbock's disease
    controversies concerning 72
    procedures 72
    radial shortening 72
    stages of progression 72
    ulnar lengthening in 72
    ulnar variance in 72
Knee 153–68
    anterior cruciate ligament injuries 155–6
    anterior pain 153–4
    arthroplasty 160–3
        after tuberculosis 161
        after unicondylar arthroplasty 161
        following failed tibial osteotomy 161
        in rheumatoid arthritis 165
        infection 162–3
    biomechanics 154–5
    discoid lateral meniscus 166
    in cerebral palsy 22
    ligament instability 155–6
    magnetic resonance imaging 154
    meniscal cysts 168
    osteoarthritis 158–63
    osteonecrosis 163–4
    popliteal cysts 167
    reflex sympathetic dystrophy 166
    replacement in haemophilic arthropathy 40
    rheumatoid arthritis 164–5

synovectomy 164–5
tuberculosis 161
unicompartmental replacement 159

Leg-length discrepancies 114, 115
Leg lengthening, callotasis method 115
Legg–Calve–Perthes' disease 123
Legg–Perthes' disease 124
Limb lengthening. See Leg lengthening;
    Lower limb
Low back pain
    after excision of lumbar disc 89
    assessment of 85
    clinical studies 86
    epidemiology 86
    epidural injections 88
    facet joint injection in 93
    manipulative treatment 88
    medical treatment 88
    psychological distress 86
    rehabilitation 86
Lower limb
    achondroplasia 46
    arthrodeses in haemophilia 40
    length discrepancy 114, 116
    lengthening 116
        Ilizarov technique 116
        in achondroplastic patients 115
        Wagner method 115
    partial physeal arrest 117
Lumbar canal stenosis in Paget's disease of
    bone 20
Lumbar disc disease 84–94
    chemonucleolysis in 92
Lumbar disc herniation 89
Lumbar disc lesions, arachnoiditis in 91
Lumbar disc prolapse in adolescence 94
Lumbar disc protrusion
    diagnosis of 87
    microsurgical treatment 90
Lumbar disc surgery, vascular injuries in 91
Lumbar discectomy 89
Lumbar disease, discography 87
Lumbar facet arthrosis syndrome 83
Lumbar instability 93
    presentation and radiological features 94
Lumbar intervertebral-disc disease, surgical
    management of 88
Lumbar intervertebral joints, torsion 85
Lumbar laminectomy 90
Lumbar nerve root, bony entrapment of 93
Lumbar spinal canal 89
Lumbar spinal nerve root canals 84
Lumbar spinal osteotomy in ankylosing
    spondylitis 34
Lumbar spine
    internal fixation 94
    postoperative MR imaging 87
Lumbar disc lesions 89